READY, SET, GO!:

YOUR ROADTRIP TO WELLNESS

A Travel Guide to Making Lifelong Lifestyle Changes for a Happier and Healthier You!

ALLIE LOWE

NATIONAL BOARD-CERTIFIED
HEALTH AND WELLNESS COACH

DISCLAIMER

The advice and strategies found within may not be suitable for every situation. This work is sold with the understanding that neither the author nor the publisher is to be held responsible for the results accrued from the advice in this book.

Ready, Set, Go!:
Your Roadtrip to Wellness

ISBN: 979-8-9850934-0-7

Contents

Forward **3**

Introduction **7**

WELCOME **13**

- A JOURNEY BEGINS WITH A SINGLE STEP 13
- WHO IS ALLIE LOWE? WHY SHOULD I TRUST HER ADVICE? 16
- WHAT TO EXPECT 21
- SEIZE THE DAY – THE TIME IS NOW! 26
- REFRAMING “GETTING HEALTHY” INTO A ROAD TRIP TO WELLNESS 29
- PLANNING YOUR ROAD TRIP 34

PREPARING FOR THE ROAD TRIP **39**

- WHAT IS WELLNESS? WHERE EXACTLY AM I GOING? 39
- POSITIVE MINDSET 43

YOU ARE HERE 57

- KNOWING AND HONORING YOURSELF 58
- RECOGNIZE AND USE YOUR STRENGTHS 61
- UNDERSTAND HOW YOU WORK 65
- SELF-ASSESSMENT 68
- SETTING YOUR VISION 75

DESTINATIONS 81

- FUNCTIONAL MEDICINE 82
- BREAKING IT INTO DAY TRIPS 87
- PRIORITIZING YOUR ITINERARY 107
- STAGES OF BEHAVIORAL CHANGE 108

WHAT TO PACK 121

- ESSENTIAL ITEMS FOR SUCCESS 122
- PACKING CHECKLIST 166

WHAT TO LEAVE BEHIND 177

- RIGIDITY – STRATEGY VS. PLANNING 179
- TIME MANAGEMENT – FINDING TIME VS. MAKING TIME 181
- OUTCOME ATTACHMENT – IT'S NOT THE DESTINATION, IT'S THE JOURNEY 184

ROAD MAPS **187**

- THE VISION 188
- DECISIONAL BALANCE 194
- BEHAVIORAL GOALS 197
- SMART GOALS 201
- YOUR DAILIES JOURNAL 208

EMBARKING ON YOUR JOURNEY **215**

- DEALING WITH UNCERTAINTY 216
- ENJOYING THE JOURNEY 220
- BECOMING YOUR OWN ROAD GUIDE 221

RETURNING HOME **225**

- EMBRACING FEAR AND FRUSTRATION 228
- THE ETERNAL TRAVELER 232

ABOUT THE AUTHOR **239**
ACKNOWLEDGMENTS **243**
RESOURCES FOR THE READER **247**

- WITHIN THIS BOOK 247
- OUTSIDE THIS BOOK 249
- RECOMMENDED READING 249

BIBLIOGRAPHY **251**

Dedication

This is for you! By picking up this book, you are acknowledging that you have choices in your life and that you can always choose to change your existence into something you want it to be.

I hope this book will inspire and motivate you to make the most meaningful road trip of your life—destination: health and wellness. I invite you to visualize, discover, and explore new alternative options to make your life as content and valuable as I know it can be.

Happy travels!

Forward

From the first time I met Allie over fourteen years ago, I knew she was a smart and inspirational woman I wanted to be my friend. She had all the qualities of a healthy, approachable, and fitness-minded individual that I, myself, aspired to be. As she changed careers from one of frequent travel and recruiting, to a more balanced one as a health coach, functional medicine practitioner, and yoga therapist, I saw her find her true calling and really blossom into a wonderful leader in our wellness community.

I remember when she had the idea for this book. She was ready to share with more than just her clients, many of whom I have referred to her and witnessed them excel with her help. She was focused on reaching out to those who felt stuck in their wellness journey and did not know or have the means to hire a personal coach. Her positive attitude and personal experience on her own path to wellness brings the reader closer to her and allows them to feel that their own speed bumps are not failures, but rather common when starting something new.

As a doctor of chiropractic, I know I can send a client to Allie or give them her book and they will be in good hands to help them reach their full potential. While I can help clients with physical pain, improving functional movement and nutrition, along with wellness adjustments, this is done with more of an authoritative style. As a health and wellness coach, Allie is a supportive guide and mentor who empowers you to take responsibility for your personal wellness goals. She can help with stress management, sleep habits, mind-body, and positive psychological interventions. She does so in a format that is similar to a travel guide. Allowing the reader to figure out their own goals, roadblocks, and behavioral choices, and tailoring an individualized road map to meet her clients' needs. Her style fulfills an important role with her clients to develop strategies that enact real, lasting lifestyle changes.

This road map will help guide you in the right direction. I am thrilled to be able to recommend it to my patients.

—Lindsay Broderick, D.C.

Dr. Broderick is board-certified and licensed in Long Beach, California. She specializes in spine and extremity joint pain reduction and management, nutrition, sport and fitness conditioning, post-injury rehabilitation, post-isometric relaxation (PIR) muscle work, myofascial release, and functional biomechanics with a focus on preventative medicine and wellness care. She has advanced training in diversified musculoskeletal adjustments, nutrition, and neuromuscular re-education. She founded Life Choice Chiropractic in 2011, which is one of Long Beach's premiere chiropractic offices. Her motto is, "Healthy by choice, not by chance!" Her office tailors their chiropractic and holistic care to the unique needs of each patient. They know that health comes from within and is much more than simply being pain-free.

Introduction

I'll bet you've wanted to improve your health for a long time. You've probably even taken a few steps in the right direction, and maybe a few steps back. Perhaps you have some goals in mind but haven't started on your journey to wellness because you just aren't sure how to begin. Yet you know, deep down, it's time to commit.

The reality is many people want to get moving on their path to becoming healthier and feeling better. But not many find the directions to get healthy and stay that way. After all, it's not always an easy route. Some common obstacles like not knowing what to eat, difficulty figuring out what kind of exercise is best, and not having enough time to practice self-care can get in the way of progress. But these are challenges that every person faces at one point or another. How do some people break through those roadblocks while others don't? What's the missing piece?

Health coaches empower their clients to create a plan (or a road map) that will help them change their habits, reach their goals, and thrive. In our world today, there may not be anything more important. You want to improve the way you feel. You want to change your relationship with food. You are ready to feel your best and have tried to go it alone, but have gone off course, gotten lost, and felt frustrated. Many people have had health goals and have experienced some success, but many of those have also had trouble navigating through the roadblocks and find it difficult to create a sustainable strategy and be consistent. If you have begun to explore becoming a healthier version of you and need support and guidance for your journey, this book is for you. Whether you want to get from point A to point B or reach a wellness goal, understanding your journey will more likely empower your efforts.

I have been a health professional and part of the wellness industry since 1995. I grew up in the world of holistic wellness as the daughter of a chiropractor, so I guess my journey into this line of work was inevitable. I built a successful, functional medicine practice, serving clients throughout the United States. During my studies in the functional medicine coaching field, I had the privilege of meeting and collaborating with some incredible practitioners. I am grateful to have met and worked alongside Allie Lowe—a savvy and talented professional with a brilliant mind, but more importantly, a loving and inspiring coach.

When Allie asked me to write this introduction, I immediately said, "Yes, of course!" The world needs the information that is contained in the pages of this book—the book that shares the essentials for being successful on a journey to wellness. As Allie perfectly details in this book, you are "traveling" to wellness, and the trip must be individualized for each person. Viewing this experience as a road trip is such an interesting and unique concept! Road trips are usually much more fun and adventurous than giving up sugar or adopting an exercise habit. When viewed through this perspective, you can make this transition much more enjoyable and longer lasting.

There are many books on wellness, but I have never seen one that reframes the desire to be healthier by teaching how to create a road trip to wellness. Allie will help you decide which essential items you must pack, how to map out your journey properly, and most importantly, how to enjoy the learning process while you embark upon your trip. If you are holding this book in your hands now, read on! Inside are the answers you've been looking for. You are ready to get healthy. You are ready to begin your road trip to wellness. Your journey begins with this book. It's time to go!

—Kate Motz, Functional Medicine Coach, NBC-HWC

Kate Motz is a National Board-certified functional medicine coach and the founder of Integrative Wellness Advisors, where she has helped people since 1995 to create sustainable wellness plans to get healthy and stay that way. Her mission is to help individuals discover the root causes of health problems because she knows—and evidence shows—that the greatest health transformations are created and sustained when you address the root cause. Raised as the daughter of a chiropractor, Kate has lived her entire life with beliefs that a holistic approach must be applied when addressing health issues, and that chronic health problems can be fixed at any age. Kate is also a published author. You can find her book, Revolutionary Weight Loss: The Predictable Plan to Lose It for Good This Time, *on Amazon.*

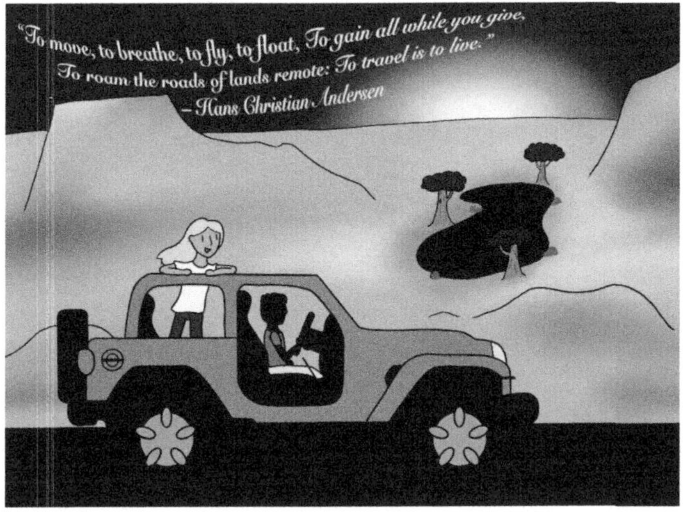
"To move, to breathe, to fly, to float, To gain all while you give,
To roam the roads of lands remote: To travel is to live."
– Hans Christian Andersen

WELCOME

BIENVENIDO – BIENVENUE –

SHALOM – HUANYING – ALOHA

WELLNESS
"A journey of a thousand miles must begin with a single step."
- Lao Tzu

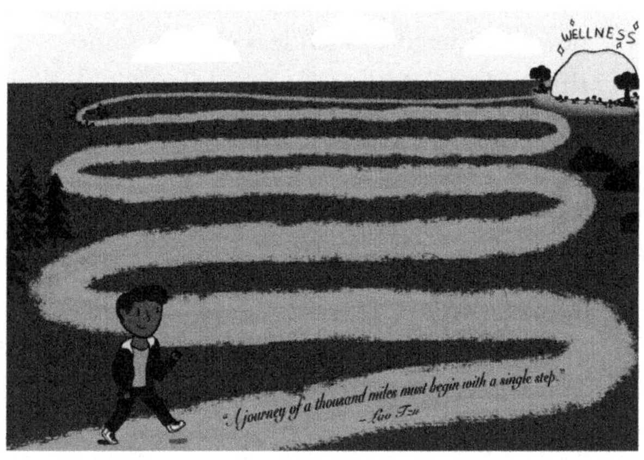

A JOURNEY BEGINS WITH A SINGLE STEP

Nine out of ten people make New Year's resolutions. . . But did you know, nine out of ten people also break their New Year's resolutions within the first week? Does this sound familiar?

> "I've got a big project for work. . . I can't possibly focus on this right now."
>
> "We have a big event coming up. . . I'll just start my diet after it's over."
>
> "I'm not sure if I really need to start exercising. I feel fine for now, and I can just go up a size."
>
> "I'm so overwhelmed. . . I get stressed out just thinking about having to do something new or different, much less give up something I love."
>
> "I'll worry about it later. . ."

All of these reasons make sense. But as my snarky daughter will point out, these reasons are why we are where we are—not feeling great, clothes not fitting right, zero energy, and wishing we were healthier.

So many of us have dreams and visions of what we'd like our lives to be. And yet, we often put them aside in the back of our minds with lesser priorities. However, when we start to feel really uncomfortable in our bodies and we can barely make it through the day, we start to wonder, "What's wrong with me?"

Why do we do this to ourselves? Why don't we act now? Why do we tolerate the way we're feeling? Many think, "I really like my life, so I don't know why I'm not happy." Time, resources, fear, and even denial are some obstacles that prevent people from getting healthier.

That was me, by the way. By the time I reached my mid-fifties, I was at the top of my game, in a great relationship, and had a prodigal daughter who constantly kept me on my toes. But something deep inside me knew that life could be better. I didn't have to be constantly in motion. I wasn't comfortable with my middle-aged spread. I knew that I could feel better. Ultimately, I knew deep down inside that I was wasting my potential. I didn't know specifically what my potential was, I just knew that I had more abilities than I was using. I was coasting.

It's easy to coast and stay in our comfort zone. There's nothing wrong with being comfortable. However, if that pesky feeling that life could be better keeps reappearing, don't we owe it to ourselves to explore what's out there? There's nothing worse than knowing that our lives could be different or better, and that we have choices we can make to live a happier and healthier existence, and still doing nothing to reach those goals.

Trust me, I've been there. Here's my story...

WHO IS ALLIE LOWE? WHY SHOULD I TRUST HER ADVICE?

Who is Allie Lowe, anyway? She's probably this perky, "healthy" person who loves kale, never eats junk food, and jumps out of bed, eager for her day to begin.

This couldn't be farther from the truth. I love my junk food, and perky is the last word you would use to describe me in the morning. To be honest, I actually stumble out of bed.

Ten years ago, I was a middle-aged single mom living with a daughter known as "The Hurricane," five animal rescues, and a very patient boyfriend. I owned a successful human resources and recruiting consultation practice, and had a busy and fun social life. Juggling life was my specialty.

For years, my doctor told me that I had the body of a thirty-year-old and, boy, did I use that to my advantage! I lived well. My daughter and I bonded over food and "essential" television like *Gilmore Girls*, *Buffy the Vampire Slayer*, and *Chopped*. I exercised only when I wanted to, and sometimes, I'd take three-month breaks and do nothing. Although my work could be stressful, I overcompensated by sleeping less, going on long runs, and eating whatever I wanted. My body and mind were exhausted, but my attitude was if I just kept going, everything else would eventually keep up.

One year during my annual check-up, my doctor paused before telling me something different from the usual, "Everything looks great!" This time, she said, "Hmmm. . . You're A1C has crept up from 4.5 to 5.9. This puts you in the prediabetic category."

Still, I was proud and in denial. I thought, "Oh, I can fix that easily. I just won't eat cake for breakfast anymore."

Umm, yeah. . . You can guess how that turned out. It wasn't as easy as I expected it to be. I struggled. I didn't realize how much sugar I was intaking. Along with the hidden sugars in my foods, I also often polished off a glass—okay, a bottle—of wine with my friends at happy hour.

It was hard to let go of sugar—it had been one of my BFFs ever since I was little. It has positive associations in my life. I bonded with my mom over cookies. I bonded with my daughter over ice cream. I bonded with myself when I finally got a night to watch Netflix and eat M&Ms mixed into my popcorn.

I tried the 80/20 rule at first, where you eat nutritiously 80% of the time and the other 20% you eat however you want. But then 80% turned into 85%, so I stopped. Then I tried eliminating sugar altogether. That lasted two days, four hours, twelve minutes, and eighteen seconds. And during that time, I wasn't fun to be around. My sudden breakup with sugar sent me into a type of withdrawal and caused me to be cranky and resentful.

Disappointingly, at the next doctor visit my A1C was even higher. Talk about rubbing salt in the wound. I was incredibly frustrated. As a highly paid consultant, someone in a wonderful relationship, surrounded by wonderful friends, and a successful parent—at least, I thought I was, although my daughter might give you a different opinion—I should have been thriving. I should have found success in my health without any trouble. So, WHY was I failing?

I turned to the experts so I could understand and fix the problem. But frankly, reading about all the science and the whys, along with the horror stories about what would happen if I wasn't able to make the necessary changes just left me sleepy, bored, and apathetic. I just wanted to know how to make the changes simply and maintain my sanity in the process.

Instead, I started doing the research myself and created a step-by-step strategy for how I would make those changes. I expanded my knowledge about functional medicine and read other people's experiences on health and wellness. I also started to meditate and practice yoga regularly, curbing my unhealthy dependance on sugar.

What I learned from this journey was that this issue was more than just a physical dependance on sugar. Several things were lacking in my life, which caused me to use sugar as a crutch. One important functional medicine concept is uncovering the root causes of your dependence. I realized there were many root causes impacting my addiction to sugar. And it wasn't just physical—it was emotional, mental, and spiritual.

That was tough to admit. From an outsider's point of view, I had the best life. And trust me, I played it to the hilt, because when you're the result of Asian parents, you're taught that everything must appear positive on the outside. I learned how to carry this out well, but I didn't know what to do with everything I was stuffing down. Inside, I was lost. I realized my busyness was just a distraction for things that I didn't want to face. I was having a midlife crisis and struggling to find my purpose and place in the world.

Going through this experience and clearing away my denial led me to coaching programs in functional medicine, positive psychology, meditation, and yoga. I had finally found something that brought me as much joy as sugar did, and in a much healthier way.

I spent the time to dig deep and understand what my dependence was really about. At first, I was frustrated with myself for not just getting it. But then I realized, this is all part of the process, part of the experience. Once I understood more about myself, I was able to change my story and figure out how to get what I really wanted with my life. I created and recreated strategies, took three steps forward and, sometimes, four steps back—it's a good thing I like doing the cha-cha!

My third visit to the doctor was the charm! I managed to reduce my A1C from 5.9 to 5.0. My doctor was thrilled. She encouraged me to get my functional medicine coaching credential so she could refer patients to me. With my knowledge and personal experience, I could be the perfect coach to help others through this common life struggle.

To say I conquered my sugar dependence is an understatement. Not only was I able to decrease my sugar intake, but I was also able to find out more about myself—what made me tick, what got me excited, what did and didn't work. And I didn't just apply this to decreasing my A1C—I applied this to my whole life! I was a caterpillar who finally morphed into a butterfly.

I've been taking what I learned from this experience and applying it to my clients' journeys. I'm excited to say it's worked for them too. As a result, many of them have encouraged me to write this book so even more people can try my methods. I'm sharing this information in hopes that it will inspire everyone to conquer their old bad habits and create new healthy ones. It just takes getting out of your comfort zone, some planning, and a little discipline. These are all things that I thought I was terrible at but found, with a little help. I could excel at each.

The concept is more than cutting something from your diet or getting on the treadmill every day. For something to really stick, we must dig deep. My coaching approach with my clients is to take the time to understand and celebrate who we are. From there, we can discover our strengths and use them to make the life that we desire.

Understanding who we are and what we can accomplish allows us to be vulnerable and accepting of our shortcomings, enabling us to come up with strategies that can help us navigate the difficult times. We each need to narrow our focus and eliminate the stories that aren't serving us anymore. Embrace the unknown and recognize that you have the power to change things. These are the actions that will lead you down the path of wellness!

I started coaching because I've met so many people who have unfulfilled dreams and sit idly on untapped potential, just like I did. My hope is that you read this book and are inspired to make small and gradual changes in your lifestyle, eliminating the risks and living your life to your fullest potential.

WHAT TO EXPECT

I want you to think of this as a road trip. If you accept me as your guide, I plan to make this journey an adventure! Fun fact: one of the things I like to do when I have the "travel bug," but can't travel—remember 2020?—is read through travel books. I love learning about the history and background of the places I want to visit. I like knowing how different each area is, the highlights of the culture, and what to expect. I appreciate the recommendations about what to pack and what to leave behind, and I count on the maps to help me understand where I am. I also enjoy exploring the souvenirs that I might take with me and treasure as precious memories of where I've been and how far I've come even years after my journey.

This is why I chose to write this book like a road trip guide to help you on your journey. I want to help you figure out what you already have, what you need to cultivate, and what to expect during your trip to wellness. I've included my own experiences and even some of my clients (with their permission, of course!) so you can understand what your own journey might be like.

In the end, what you choose to use and what you choose to discard is your decision to make, and yours alone. I want to stress that not everything in here will work for you. The beauty of this book will be to inspire you, learn more about yourself, and discover what kind of traveler you are. Once you understand this, you'll be able to plan your own unique road trip to wellness.

YOUR ROAD TRIP TO WELLNESS

Preparing for the Road Trip – This chapter is all about wellness and why it's important to have a positive mindset from the beginning. In this section, I will cover what wellness truly is, help you see why you would be interested in it, and aid you in recognizing the benefits. I will discuss how you can be successful in your own wellness and what it will take. I will offer reasons why having a positive mindset is helpful when you start making healthy changes, and what the key factors are in successfully cultivating this mindset. I will also discuss where positive psychology and mindfulness originate.

You Are Here – This chapter will help you understand who you are in this present moment. I know this seems silly, but the truth is many of us don't take the time to understand where we're starting from. Who are you? How can you honor the complex individual that you are? What works for you? What do you want out of life? Best of all, what are your strengths and how you can leverage them while going after your health goals, or any goals for that matter?

Understanding why you want something is one of the key factors to getting it. I find that people often skip this step, and when things get challenging or they run into obstacles, it's very easy to just quit. Carefully understanding and creating a vivid vision will help you stay on track. Taking the time to understand your "why" is a key factor for your successful and wonderful journey! I also will guide you to create a unique vision board that will remind you daily to keep your vision alive.

Destinations – This chapter will inspire you with ideas of what type of lifestyle changes you'd like to make. "Wait a minute, Coach Allie. I don't need to learn this stuff. I already know where I want to go. I want to lose my 'COVID 15.' Just point me in that direction!"

While this is a great starting point, losing a few pounds can be short term, and it's only a tiny piece of the puzzle to wellness. Let's say you lose the weight. Do you feel satisfied or always hungry? Do you find that you gain the weight back quickly if you slip up just a little bit? Are you always tired? Are you constantly stressed? Do you feel isolated?

Wellness encompasses many different areas besides just dropping pounds. Don't skip this step on your journey to wellness and success. In this chapter, you'll learn about all the possible areas (i.e.: destinations) that you may want to explore through a functional medicine lens. With this approach, you'll be able to achieve overall wellness faster *and* have a longer lasting impact. Don't worry, I'll cover what functional medicine is and why this is becoming our new approach to deal with health issues. We'll also take the time to learn how to break down your destinations into easy and attainable "day trip" goals.

We'll discuss how to prioritize your itinerary with a Wellness Wheel and help you understand the different behavioral change stages (baby steps rule!). So many times, we try to jump from level one to level four, only to drop back to level two (oh my gosh, why am I going *backward*?). This is known as the cha-cha-cha of adopting a healthy habit. Hopefully, some understanding of these changes will help you do a little less dancing and a little more forward momentum.

What to Pack – This chapter will cover the essential items you need for success! How will you show up? How can you be mindful and incorporate a centered and peaceful approach to your goals? How can you build resiliency when it gets tough and increase your self-efficacy and self-confidence so you feel you can take on the world? How can you engage your world to help support you with your goals? I'll help you create a packing checklist that will ensure you'll have every possible skill you need. We'll talk about how you can measure and cultivate these valuable skills to help you on your road trip.

What to Leave Behind – For you over-packers (formerly, me!), this chapter will help guide you on the things you need to let go of. There are some common pitfalls that we all encounter and, hopefully, this will make your travels a lot smoother and lighter! Sometimes, when we have too much baggage, it's hard to find the room to take in new information. Leave your rigidity, stress, and outcome attachment behind, and take the cannoli (I couldn't resist!).

Road Maps – This chapter will provide tools for you to use during your road trip. These tools will help you plan and track your progression on your journey. I'll help you sort out your priorities, flesh out the pros and cons, and measure your readiness. One of the most valuable things I offer my clients is how to break down that wonderful vision into smaller behavioral goals. You'll learn how to make SMART goals and track your daily progress. Many of my clients want the results *now* (Veruca Salt, anyone?), and if they don't see them, they tend to get discouraged really easily. The ability to see how far you've come from day one will help you understand that the value is in the process, or the journey. This will keep you moving forward.

Embarking on Your Journey – This chapter will help you understand if you have everything you need, and if you've gotten rid of what you don't need. It's also about finding enjoyment on this road trip and carving out your unique experience.

You will become your own expert road guide and master the deliberate practice and flow.

Returning Home – Finally, this chapter will talk about how we can save our souvenirs and just how much this journey can change who we are. This will be exhilarating, scary, frustrating, and life changing. If you're anything like me, you'll want more. We'll talk about how we can keep traveling forward forever!

This book is written purposely as a road trip guide. In a sense, your journey to a healthy life is a road trip—perhaps the biggest one of your life. Making healthy changes to your lifestyle can be overwhelming, confusing, and frustrating at first. But breaking it down might make your journey a little less painful and more of an adventure. My hope after you finish this book is to be inspired to meet your health goals successfully. As with traveling, you will be a different person at the conclusion, learn how to get out of your comfort zone, and take home new and beneficial experiences that you will keep forever.

SEIZE THE DAY – THE TIME IS NOW!

> *Seize the day, take hold of it, and make it whatever you want!*
>
> —Jessica Sorensen

This has never been more true, especially now that we've lived through 2020. In just one year, we've experienced a pandemic, racial unrest, and a whole different way of living.

During a conference call with my fellow wellness coaches, we started talking about how underlying conditions had such a big impact on this insidious virus. According to a recent modeling study by The Lancet Global Health organization, one in five people has at least one underlying condition such as cancer, chronic kidney disease, COPD (chronic obstructive pulmonary disease), Down syndrome, heart conditions, weakened immune system, obesity (defined by having a body mass index over $30kg/m^2$), pregnancy, sickle cell disease, smoking, type 2 diabetes mellitus, and more.

Many of these conditions are chronic and lifestyle driven. In the United States alone, four out of ten adults have two or more chronic health conditions. Chronic disease is the leading cause of death and disability. It's no surprise, then, that wellness is such a big movement nowadays, especially when strains of COVID impact people with underlying conditions the worst. And even if you're lucky enough to avoid this virus while having a chronic issue, I'm going to guess that you may be still struggling. And let's not forget aging—our bodies aren't keeping up with our busy lives. We can't control COVID, what we did in the past, or the fact that we are aging, but we can make the choice to start today to positively influence our lifestyle and take control of our own lives.

The people I work with are ready to change their lives. Usually, this isn't their first time around. They've tried to make these changes on their own and had discouraging experiences. The ones who have been successful at the start are now struggling to maintain their new healthy habits. Some people are in great pain and suffering from chronic diseases, and some are in a panic because their doctor has informed them that they will be dead in five years due to their cholesterol and blood sugar levels.

If any of these stories resonate with you, you are in good company!

> "I've been successful all my life. I've got a great career, family, and life! But lately, I've lost all my energy. It's just going from one thing to another. I'm so stressed out!"

> "I just got back from the doctor, and he told me that my cholesterol has gone through the roof! I always thought I was healthy, but now he's telling me I'm at risk for heart attacks and diabetes. Then he rushed out of the room to see his other patients. What about me? After that bombshell, what do I do now?"

> "I'm a professional dieter. I try the newest diet, lose weight, and then gain it all back again when I start eating regular food. I think I'm even heavier now than when I started. Why can't I stick to something?"

> "I'm pretty happy with my life, but I feel like something is missing. I have all this potential inside me that's not being used. I start things, but never finish them, and now I'm starting to feel depressed. I know I can feel better, I just don't know where to start."

The key to increasing our wellness is changing our lifestyle and giving up our stories that no longer serve us. We might have to do things that we never thought we'd do (a great example for me is drinking green juice). When we open our minds, it will change the way we look at things. Sometimes, this can be exhilarating! Other times, this can be scary. If you're feeling both, let me assure you that this is completely normal. Changing your lifestyle is DIFFICULT. Not only will you lose something that you've been clinging to all your life, but you will also have to bravely venture out of your comfort zone.

REFRAMING "GETTING HEALTHY" INTO A ROAD TRIP TO WELLNESS

If you want to achieve wellness, the truth is you will have to go on a journey. If you think about it, you take journeys each time you're in unknown situations. Merriam-Webster defines a journey as "something suggesting travel or passage from one place to another." Your world is always changing and you're making journeys every day, whether between physical locations or mental ones.

When you take a road trip, you explore different paths to reach your final destination. You expose yourself to new places, cultures, and alternate ways of living. Your wellness journey is very much like a road trip, and you will experience similar situations. There will be wonderful lessons along the way on your wellness journey. For example, I learned that Swiss chard is not my favorite taste in a smoothie and filling up on veggies tones down my snacking habit.

Let's make this journey fun by reframing your desire to be healthier into a road trip to wellness. Instead of a cumbersome, negative approach, let's look at this as a time for you to explore, discover who you are, and determine how you want to live. It's an adventure!

When you take a trip, there are some expectations that will never be met. Does this mean that your whole trip is ruined? I hope not! As a well-worn traveler, I have found that there are always hiccups while traveling, but as a whole, most trips have positive memories. Even some disastrous trips have positive memories because you bonded with your travel mates over how bad the circumstances were. Take, for example, the camping trip where it rained cats and dogs, and then the sun came out the day you were leaving. It might not have been the most fun situation in the moment, but I bet you look back on it with laughter and fondness.

Just like any vacation, there's an element of the unknown. It's also important to note that every journey is individualized and there's no "one trip fits all" that will work for everyone.

You will have to decide where you want to go and understand why you want to go in the first place. Many of you may have planned your vacations before and know they have a very specific goal in mind—you want to relax, you want to learn, you want to take good pictures. Your journey to wellness is just like that. You can't see the whole world at once, and the same is true when you're trying to be healthier. You're not going to get healthy overnight or be able to take care of everything with just one trip. And while spontaneity and surprises are wonderful elements of a trip, for it to be successful, you'll need to do some sort of preparation to have a rough (and flexible) plan in place. It's quite a balance—sketching out a foundation while allowing enough flexibility to deal with obstacles, unforeseen events, and well, to just have fun. It's harder than it may seem, but I'm here to help!

Traveling changes you. Through your experiences, you'll start to see things from a different perspective and better understand yourself. You will learn who you truly are and what you want out of life. You can also see how good your present life is and feel grateful. I think it's safe to say that most of us travel because we want to have a change of scenery or a change of pace. We want something to be different—to have a different experience or to feel a different way.

Unlike a typical vacation that usually has a single destination, a road trip has several destinations on the journey. The focus is on the stops along the way. You have more flexibility with road trips than destination vacations. For example, if you enjoy a place on one of your stops, you can choose to stay there for as long as you want. You could also change your mode of transportation, lodging, places to see, and who you travel with.

I like the idea of a goal becoming a destination. You may start out with one primary objective and, while you're on your way, discover other destinations that you want to explore as well. Let's say your goal/destination is losing ten pounds. On your way to losing ten pounds, you'll discover a food plan that will work for you. You'll get interested in a new exercise that doesn't necessarily feel like exercise—maybe tennis. You may also want to spend more quality time with your family. Maybe tennis is something that appeals to everyone and is, therefore, something you can all do together—not just for exercise, but for entertainment. You find that playing tennis every week has strengthened your relationships as well as help you to get moving. It's helps you sleep better. You discover that the combination of weekly exercise, a new food plan, better relationships, and enough sleep has decreased your stress level. And the benefits just keep rolling in. Your primary destination just led you to four other destinations. Now that's a road trip I want to take!

I've been coaching for over five years and have helped my clients go on their own road trips to wellness. I decided to write this book because I often talk to people who want to make healthy changes, but don't know where to start. I find that this is rather common, and I want to help as many people as I can. These people are overwhelmed with too much information, feeling frustrated because of their past attempts and failures, and don't know if they have what it takes to truly be successful.

I'd like to volunteer to be your road guide through this trip. In this book, I'll be sharing concepts and tips from my holistic specialties—functional medicine, positive psychology, yoga, and meditation. These four disciplines will be able to take some of the load off the overwhelm and frustration you may have experienced in the past. I don't want to overwhelm you even more, so please note that we'll briefly talk about the basic concepts. For those of you who want more, I'll leave a resource page so you can dig a little deeper on your own (and I hope you do!).

The time for making positive changes is NOW. There's no better time than right now to start this trip! Don't push your health and happiness aside anymore. Everyone has what it takes to be successful in making healthy changes to their lives, and you will be glad you did when you see how much it can affect your whole life for the better. Imagine yourself letting go of that excess baggage of reasons, bad habits, and the things that prevent you from living the best life that you can. Explore your choices and customize a way of life that will help you thrive. Know that you can live a life that you choose because you know what you are capable of.

I'm beyond excited for you! You'll learn so much about yourself, what motivates you, and what works for you, and all of this will set you up for long-term success. My hope is that once you've taken your first wellness road trip, you'll be back for more. Continually taking these trips year after year will only benefit you!

Do this for yourself. Stop waiting. Seize the day.

PLANNING YOUR ROAD TRIP

In our house, there is a continuous debate on how to prepare for a road trip. I'm a planner—I plan out each stop, where we're going to stay, choose interesting attractions to visit, and most importantly, I plan the food (c'mon, you haven't lived until you've tried Wisconsin cheese curds or Brooklyn hot dogs!). My partner is the complete opposite. He loves to take detours and prefers living "in the moment." Discovering an unknown place, taking his time to photograph yet another waterfall in Iceland, and taking a day of rest are his elements of a perfect trip. I hate to admit it, but sometimes he may be right.

When taking your road trip to wellness, it's important to keep in mind that there needs to be a balance between planning and flexibility. If you want to make healthy changes in your life, you *will* need a strategy. It's not enough to say you want to be better at exercising. You have to schedule it into your day, or else you run the risk of not actually following through. Hope is not a good strategy. A plan will guide and prepare you for the work that needs to be done.

However, becoming obsessive with planning (yep, that can be me!), can make you miss the best parts of life or even cause you to fail at your ultimate goal. Let's say you decided to run a marathon in six months. The first month goes really well, and you're hitting your target miles. But then work gets busy, and now there's wear and tear on your knee from running so much. Running a marathon may not be your goal anymore. In fact, rigidly sticking to this plan would do more harm than good. It would hurt your body and sacrifice your recovery.

But does that mean you failed or that it's time to give up? Absolutely, not! This is where flexibility comes in to save the day. Stepping back to fully understand *why* you want to run a marathon will help you find different options. Did you want to lose weight? Did you want to run off your stress? There is more than just one way to accomplish your ultimate goal. Remaining fluid and flexible will help you to achieve your "end game," whatever it may be. Don't give up on what you really want, just look for another road that could take you there. And who knows, maybe you'll find something that you love even more than running.

Let's say you made plans to do a yoga class with your friend at the new studio in town. Then your kids got sick, you got that extra project at work that you've been hoping for, and—*whoops!*—now you have a sore throat. Time to "go with the flow." Instead of going to the studio, you squeeze in an on-demand online restorative class with your friend before an early bedtime. You can do this by pressing "play" at the same time in your respective homes. This will help to hold you both accountable to actually follow through.

This reminds me of when I was in Paris planning to visit the Eiffel Tower. It rained *chats et chiens.* Instead, we switched gears and found a charming café to wait out the rain. They made the best café au lait, and we had a life-changing conversation, which I probably remember more fondly than the eventual visit to the Eiffel Tower!

Starting out with a plan, but also knowing that it may change due to life is the way to go. Keeping an open mind and focusing on the big-picture objective will make your road trip to wellness smoother and more enjoyable. After all, it's the journey, not the destination. There will always be alternate routes to get to the ultimate destination. The traveler who can let go of their original plan and improvise when obstacles are thrown in their path will enjoy the trip much more. They'll also be more likely to find success in their journey over the traveler who needs to do it exactly as originally planned. You don't have to give up when life presents obstacles. You just have to be open to finding an alternate way to get to where you want to go.

Another thing to remember is that we're all different individuals, which means we have different skills, motivations, mindsets, timelines, and objectives. Following a Paleo diet when you're a vegetarian or going on a vegetarian diet when you're sensitive to grain is a recipe for disaster. You certainly can do it, but the question is how long will you *want* to do it? The changes you make should be something you can be consistent with for the rest of your life. A temporary diet is not the answer. Suffering is not the answer. I always give a knowing smile to clients who only want to stay on the diet until they lose ten pounds. Like clockwork, they always sheepishly reach out to me the next season to beg for help because—guess what—they found them again! To make lasting changes, you'll need to create something that'll work with who you are right now and stay with you for the long haul.

Honor that you're human and life happens. It doesn't mean you have to give anything up. It just means you have to plan ahead of time accordingly. With contingencies in mind, keep everything fluid and flexible, and remember that the point is to enjoy the journey, not to just get there. Life is full of many challenges and if you look at this as an adventure, I promise you, it will make it more pleasant and exciting.

Are you ready? Let's go!

PREPARING FOR THE ROAD TRIP

"The real voyage of discovery consists not in seeking new landscapes, but
in having new eyes."
–Marcel Proust

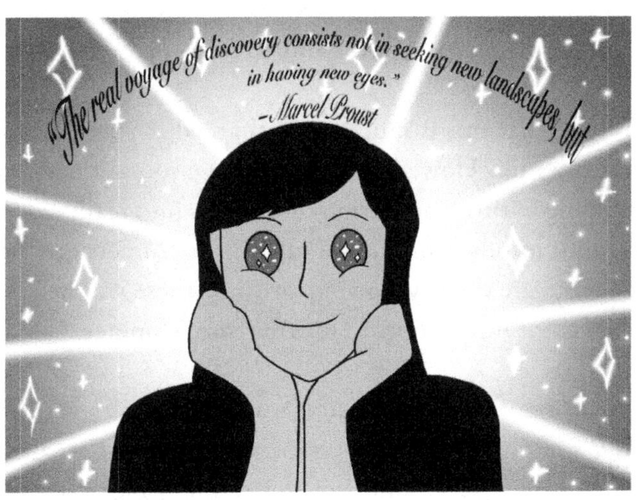

WHAT IS WELLNESS? WHERE EXACTLY AM I GOING?

As we discussed earlier, wellness is an expansive topic that covers many facets of your life. You may have picked up this book because you wanted to change your eating habits, start a regular exercise program, or get more sleep. You also may be suffering from chronic stress (aren't we all?) and you're looking for ideas to dial down your busy, chaotic life.

You've come to the right place. I'm going to take this opportunity to plant a bigger seed.

Wellness is about leading a healthy lifestyle and avoiding disease. It's also about putting your mind, body, and soul in the state of reaching its full potential. It is a committed choice to take action and change things in your life to make a positive impact in your well-being.

I realize that this is much more than what you may have signed up for. However, if you're going to use the energy and time to turn your vision of wellness into reality, opening your mindset and taking the time to understand how you work are the keys to your success. These will help you adapt to healthy habits that bring you happiness.

One of the first things you'll want to do is break down what wellness is. Here's a surprise—it doesn't mean the same thing for everyone. For some, it may mean they can fit into their high school cheerleading uniform, run a marathon without dying, jump out of bed because they're so excited for the day to start, or get right back up after being knocked down. For most of us, it's a blend of all of these.

Merriam-Webster defines wellness as, "The quality or state of being in good health especially as an actively sought goal." But my favorite definition is from the medical tab of the Free Dictionary, where it states, "A philosophy of life and personal hygiene that views health as not merely the absence of illness but the full realization of one's physical and mental potential."

There are three great nuggets in this definition.

1. **A Philosophy of Life**

   You don't have to be perfect or give up everything you love in order to be healthy. It simply means you should live a lifestyle that promotes wellness. By creating healthy habits, you will look and feel good, but this doesn't mean you can't also live life to the fullest. It just means that you want your body, mind, and spirit to be in balance, and that means choosing to live your life in a way that achieves that. Sometimes a great pecan bar or a glass of wine makes me feel great and helps me celebrate life! I won't indulge every day, but I can enjoy these things once in a while. (Don't let anyone tell you that a good pecan bar can't make your day!)

2. **Not Merely the Absence of Illness**

   You can be physically fit and still not be well if you're obsessing over what you ate last week. You can be successful in your career, but still feel isolated and empty at the end of the day. You can feel connected and successful, but barely able to get out of bed because you don't feel well physically. Are you sensing a theme here? It's all about using your full potential to find balance. Wellness is a holistic approach to ensuring that your body, mind, and soul are all in balance.

3. **Full Realization**

   This means you are making a deliberate effort, and that's where we all may fall a little bit short. If you're anything like me, I will start a new health-related goal and go full speed ahead. I do great for the first week, but then my enthusiasm starts to wane. I'll justify any slip-ups as moderation, and then it just goes downhill from there. Psychologically, this can wreak havoc on your self-esteem and self-efficacy. It can take you deeper in your self-loathing and decrease your confidence in yourself. Pretty soon, you're in that deep black hole where you feel that you just can't do anything right. Does this sound familiar? If it does, congratulations. You just admitted that you are human.

I started my wellness journey about five years ago and loved it so much that I wanted to help other people take their own journey. It's not easy, and there will be days that you just want to go back to where you were. But as you progress, something inside you will push you along. You'll start to feel better, more motivated, and adventurous. You'll start to acquire more confidence in yourself and feel at peace.

POSITIVE MINDSET

Always look on the bright side of life.

—Monty Python

If you're a *Monty Python* fan, I hope you hear the tune of one of my favorite songs in your head. Just between you and me, I hum this song before I'm about to do something that I don't particularly like doing. Why? Because as our teachers, parents, and coaches say, "Attitude is everything." It's the argument for a positive mindset.

Of course, this is easier said than done. When it comes to doing something that you've never done before or that is difficult for you, having a positive mindset will see you through. Your beliefs and the lens you see them through can make or break your journey and will determine whether you will be successful in your quest for wellness.

Have you ever dreaded a specific event? I always dreaded Monday mornings. So much so, that on Sunday nights, I would get in a funk. It felt as if I was going to a funeral, I'd be in a negative mood, and nothing could shake it. Come Monday morning, I was always right. Every single week, Monday would prove to be terrible. I always had too much to do and not enough hours in the day, and I knew I was going to fail at something or not get everything done.

But here's the thing—if you believe that things will go badly or will be awful, your mind will follow through with the negative experience over and over. It's a self-fulfilling prophecy in which your subconscious tries to keep you from attempting to do it again. In a sense, your mind is trying to protect you from harm. It listens to your emotions and goes on autopilot to ensure that you're safe from any negative experiences. It's like a helpful parent who prevents you from being adventurous because they are so focused on you being safe instead.

I had a fixed mindset toward Mondays. I believed that everything was already set in stone, and I couldn't do anything to change it—it would always be a horrible day. I was resentful and really didn't enjoy this part of my life. Mondays became just another thing to get anxious about. I worried that people around me were silently judging how poorly I was handling things. It felt like everything I did was under someone else's scrutiny.

But what if great things could happen on Mondays? What if I found opportunities to grow my business or learn something valuable? What if I was able to make it all the way through my dance class without huffing and puffing? If you *believe* good things can happen, it will open your mind and make the possibilities *real.* If you only ever view your life through a dark, negative lens, you will never discover the positive side. We sometimes get in our own way of happiness. If I never opened my mind to the positive aspects of Mondays, I would have missed out on so many opportunities!

Going through my coaching training helped me reset my fixed mindset and move toward growth. I had to let go of my anxiety and resentment. I had to get comfortable with not knowing everything. I had to start believing in myself—I have the ability to learn and develop skills that will get me to where I want to go. Now I approach each challenge and new experience as opportunities to learn and grow and having this change of attitude has changed my life!

Some of my clients have tried to make healthy lifestyle changes and had disastrous experiences. Unfortunately, this has left them with doubts and anxiety. They're understandably resistant to trying again. I was told point-blank by one of my clients that the only reason why he was reaching out to me was because his wife wouldn't stop nagging him to do something about his cholesterol. In his mind, he'd already tried a million times before and he was resigned to his fate—he'd already given up.

Some other clients had issues with their self-efficacy—a person's belief that they can be successful when carrying out a particular task. Low self-efficacy can be the worst sort of sabotage because it leads you to believe that what you're trying to do is harder than it really is, and even unattainable. Believing in yourself and your ability to accomplish your goals provides a strong momentum and helps you become more resilient and motivated. It gives you a higher chance at success. Without self-efficacy, not only will you hate your journey, but you'll also convince yourself to give up before you even leave home.

With some hard work and commitment, I was able to guide my clients into a growth mindset, teaching them that mistakes aren't setbacks, but merely opportunities for them to try new things and learn new skills. Through this change of view, my clients were able to transition into a more positive mindset and increase their self-efficacy.

POSITIVE PSYCHOLOGY

I know I promised not to be too "sciency." I will keep this introduction brief, but I need to discuss one of the newest movements within psychology because I believe it will help you in your journey.

Positive psychology is a branch of psychology that focuses on strengths and building a good life through positive experiences, states, and traits. It nurtures qualities such as optimism, resilience, gratitude, and compassion. According to Dr. Christopher Peterson's article on the Psychology Today website, the official definition is, "Positive psychology is the scientific study of what makes life most worth living" (Peterson, "Positive Psychology").

Dr. Martin Seligman, one of the pioneers of positive psychology, started using this scientific method to explore and explain why happy people were, well, happy. His research uncovered that the most satisfied and upbeat people were those who had discovered and exploited their unique combination of signature strengths (I'll touch more on this later. . .). This quest started when he noticed in the course of his study that some dogs would not quit trying to achieve their goal, proving that helplessness was not a learned trait. He later connected this with human depression.

According to Seligman, you can experience three levels of happiness:

1. **Pleasure and Gratification** – "Yay, I get to go to the movies!"

2. **Using Your Strengths** – "Wow, I was able to figure out how to solve that problem today!"

3. **Meaning and Purpose** – "I love being a mother. Making my kids feel safe and secure makes me happy!"

In a landmark speech with the American Psychological Association (APA), Dr. Seligman declared that psychology needed to shift its core study to what makes people *happy*. There was too much emphasis on the causes of mental illnesses, and not enough focus on what we're good at or how to improve that aspect of our lives.

PERMA

An important positive psychology concept is PERMA, a model that describes five core elements of psychological well-being and happiness. This concept highlights the following elements that can help people work toward a life of fulfillment, happiness, and meaning.

P – POSITIVE EMOTIONS

Positive emotions are the most direct connection to happiness and wellness. It's easy and even pleasant to work if you have positive emotions. This consists of more than just smiling and whistling while you work ("Heigh-ho, heigh-ho. . .")—it's a mindset and the ability to remain optimistic. Optimism is a powerful tool. It can help you work through the daily tasks (albeit, boring) and help you push through obstacles and challenges by moving you forward with the hope of eventual outcomes.

When I was training for my yoga teacher credential, we were encouraged to try different studios and types of classes. In my enthusiasm, I unknowingly signed up for a hot yoga class. My past experience with hot yoga was at a Bikram studio ten years ago. The room was heated to ninety-five-plus degrees. I tend to be claustrophobic, and it did not go well for me in that class. When I start to remember that experience, my body starts to send panicky sensations.

Imagine my dread when I willed myself to show up for the class this time and noticed that people from the previous class were sweating buckets as they walked out. The teacher knew I was new to the studio and made a special effort to welcome me, but it made me feel cornered. The option to silently leave the class was gone after this greeting.

I realized that this experience could go two ways. I could continue to let my mind and emotions cause me to believe

I would have an unpleasant time like last time, turning this class into another negative experience. Or I could summon my optimism to help me through the next hour. Fortunately, I chose the latter, and it affected me not only during the class, but forever afterward.

I decided to use my past experience as information and approached this class with care. I purposely used half my strength rather than pushing myself too hard. I knew from last time that my body would have to compensate for the heat. I kept my mind open to the new experience and things that I might learn.

Long story short, I got a lot out of that class. In fact, I started going regularly because I discovered that I liked the challenge. It empowered me, and I felt resilient and strong afterwards. If I had gone into this with anxiety and pessimism, I would have never found that resilience or gained the ability to rise to the challenge. I would've never been able to increase my confidence and my self-esteem.

Bear in mind that having a positive mindset doesn't mean you need to be happy 100% of the time. That's unrealistic and inauthentic. Rather, it simply means you need to find acceptance of the past regardless of how bad it was and keep faith that things will work out somehow. Doing so can help you avoid the spiral of negative feelings.

As we've all experienced, negative feelings can be incredibly discouraging, make you feel stuck, or even cause you to give up. When those moments come, hang on tight. Start smiling because, believe it or not, science is now proving the "fake it until you make it" theory is real. Recent research has shown that "a smile spurs a chemical reaction in the brain, releasing certain hormones such as dopamine and serotonin" (Spector, "Smiling"). These hormones trick your brain into believing you're happy, which then creates true feelings of happiness. Positive emotions can boost your body's resistance, build your immunity, and reduce your stress, so keep faking it till you make it!

E – ENGAGEMENT

We all find enjoyment in different things, but is there something in your life that can keep you engaged for hours and hours? Something that causes you to become so engrossed and absorbed that time flies by? This is known as the "flow"—blissful immersion into a task or activity. Not only do these activities give us joy, but they also stretch our intelligence, skills, and emotional capabilities. Finding something that engages you will help you achieve a healthy sense of well-being, fulfillment, and satisfaction in life.

There are so many people who are on autopilot. They're stuck in a life that they thought was safe, but instead they find themselves dreading each day. There's no joy, there's no engagement. It's just day after day of putting out fires and going through the motions.

I've seen this in some of my clients in their approach to their jobs, families, and life. In an attempt to make up for their misery, many will indulge in unhealthy habits like overeating, drinking too much alcohol, or zoning out on the TV. Don't get me wrong, life can be monotonous at times for all of us. There are always going to be the drudgery duties that we hate doing. The difference is, for some of us, we know these menial tasks will lead to the life that we want (there's that optimism again!). The important factor here is forward movement.

I think it's great that you want to change a physical aspect of your life to become happier and healthier. That's a big first step! But it's also important to incorporate joy and "flow" into your daily routine. Purposely making time for a passion or hobby is equivalent to choosing to engage in life. Reconnecting to the joys and loves of your life is a way to manage life on your own terms despite the obligations and duties you might have. You can have the best of both worlds—it just requires some thought and action. What engages you? What makes you "flow"? If you're having trouble with these questions, this may be a great "destination" for you to explore. Life is too short to exist on autopilot.

R – RELATIONSHIPS

> *No man is an island entire of itself; every man is a piece of the continent.*
>
> —John Donne

Humans are social creatures, hardwired to bond and depend on each other. It's not surprising, then, that relationships are part of the wellness model of positive psychology. We need other people to make us feel safe, valued, and like we belong to something greater than ourselves.

Many people I know have worked very hard to get where they are in life. Some have even sacrificed relationships on their way to the top of the ladder. Not surprisingly, when most of them reach their fifties, even though they reached their career goals, they look around and realize that they're celebrating alone.

Often, these people come to me when they reach this point. For some, their doctor may have pushed them my way due to their high blood pressure from chronic stress. Relationships are crucial to human life—we need to feel connected. Our nervous system has a specific nerve known as the vagus nerve that plays a role in our emotion regulation, social connections, and fear response. Read that again—our bodies are physically built for social connection.

M – MEANING

I've never been a big fan of busy work. My daughter is struggling with this now that she's in her first year of college and I totally get it. How much of our life consists of busy work? Can we connect this amount of work to a greater purpose or meaning?

When I was a corporate recruiter, I fell headfirst into this trap. If I made one hundred calls a day, then I did my job. Of course, no one answered their phone, and I would usually end up leaving messages. Then the whole day would be spent playing phone tag with the hundred people I called. Not meaningful, and definitely not fulfilling.

I didn't start enjoying my work until I stopped emphasizing the number of calls that I made and started focusing on the connections instead. When I took the time to explain my purpose through an email or voicemail, and then asked enough questions to understand what my potential candidates were looking for, it created a very different context. I could see the purpose in my job, and they could see the purpose of why I was calling them. I was no longer just going through the motions; I was fulfilling a purpose.

How many of us are on autopilot and not connecting our busy lives with the meaning behind them? Are we just chasing our tails in this mad race to make more money? Talk about a slippery slope—the more we buy, the more we want. At the end of the day, no matter how much money sits in our bank accounts, how happy are we, really? When we are unhappy, we often drink and eat to make up for it or try to fill the void, and then feel terrible afterwards. This is a horrible cycle that I want to help people break!

It wasn't until I became a parent that I found some meaning in my life. I'm not saying everyone needs to be a parent to find a sense of purpose, but you do need to find something that matters to you. What is the factor for you that is more important than material wealth or good times? What will drive you toward fulfillment?

Your purpose will help to anchor you in happiness. It will guide you on your path and bring you joy. Understanding the impact of what you're doing and how you might be changing the world may help you deal with the mundane and repetitive part of your daily life. No matter where I go, I know that my purpose—my daughter—will always keep me on track.

A – ACHIEVEMENTS

> *To achieve well-being and happiness, we must look back on our lives with a sense of accomplishment: "I did it, and I did it well."*
>
> —Dr. Martin Seligman

I might be going out on the limb here, but the current trend of getting a trophy just for showing up leaves me feeling a little *meh*. You should get encouragement and support when you are moving forward, but I think to celebrate someone just for starting a program or actively participating is the opposite of helpful—it's detrimental. What happens after you get the trophy? Do you still work as hard? Will you still try to improve and push further? Or do you feel satisfied calling it a day because someone recognized your efforts? Will you just do the bare minimum again next time because that's all that is required of you?

The capital *A* in PERMA isn't just a participation trophy. It's the acknowledgment that you had a sense of accomplishment! You worked toward and achieved mastery over something that you've never done before. There's also an opportunity to relish in the moment. When you master something, it usually requires sacrifice, obstacles, and meaning.

Close your eyes and think about your last accomplishment. Grab hold of that moment and remember how it felt and how much you still appreciate that experience. What was the difference between simply showing up to class and getting a high grade?

Your achievements are yours alone. Don't compare yourself with everyone else; compare your current self to your past self. Achievements and accomplishments come from attempting, engaging, and trying something new. Push yourself a little more each time to expand your skills and knowledge. Set your own bar, enjoy that experience, and understand what it provided to you while moving forward.

By understanding what positive psychology is, your road trip to wellness should be more enjoyable. Instead of focusing on what's wrong, work to use your strengths, integrate the good and bad aspects (which help you understand and appreciate any limitations), and become the best version of yourself. Dr. Margarita Tarragona, one of the most well-known positive psychology experts, said, "We can choose to embody, bring forth, or perform different ways of being, different versions of 'who we are.'"

Can you imagine the possibilities with this concept? You can choose which version is closest to your dream. What values, commitments, and kinds of relationships do you want to have? Take control and find new meaning in your life by reframing your stories. Choose which way of being you want to be; decide *who* you want to be.

YOU ARE HERE

"A traveler without observation is a bird
without wings."
– Moslih Eddin Saadi

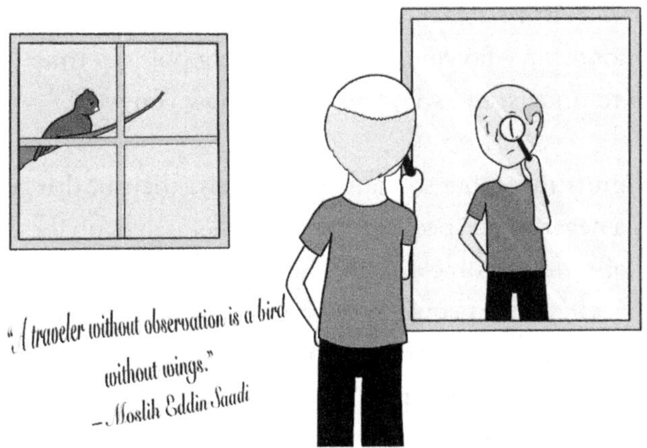

Before your trip, you need to carve out time on your calendar, assess your budget, and determine the important things and places that you want to see. You also must decide what your ultimate goal is for the trip. Is it to relax? To learn? To have an adventure? But first, let's get to know where you are starting from.

KNOWING AND HONORING YOURSELF

I have great clients. They're very determined and successful at what they do. But when they first come to me, their expectations are often low—they don't really think they need me because not much, if anything, is going to change for them. They've already tried, so what makes this any different?

Please, don't dwell on past failures and "rest on your laurels." Sometimes, no matter how determined you are, life gets in your way. Schedules, commitments, and guilt sabotage your efforts. Your first step on this road trip should be knowing and honoring who you are in this present point in time. Dig deep to understand who you are and how you work.

It's unfortunate that so many people start their health goals with a negative perspective. They beat themselves up for their lack of self-control, claim they're victims of circumstances, or that they have people in their lives who aren't supportive. There's fear in making any changes because they believe they've already given up so much. They believe it's an unattainable goal and out of their control. How successful do you think these people are in the long term?

I had a client who wanted to establish an exercise plan. She wanted to get the weight off quickly, so she committed to a running club which meant doing three-mile runs, three times a week. Sounds good, right? What she didn't realize was that while she loved running in her twenties, she was now in her forties, and running was not as enjoyable as it used to be. Now she was getting aches and pains because her body was different. She became frustrated and gave up her exercise plan within the first month. She was angry at her body and bemoaned her lack of commitment to her exercise goals. She told me, "I just gave up! I'm a loser. And to make it worse, I've gained even more weight!"

Of course, she's not a loser. She just didn't accept that things were different. What once worked for her in the past doesn't work now, and that's okay. It doesn't mean she has to give up exercise altogether, she just has to embrace who she is *now* and come up with alternative ways of exercising.

After some counsel, she decided that she wanted to try rowing. She'd never tried it before, and it was the best sport for her tweaky knee. The next month, she animatedly told me about her new friends and how strong her upper body was becoming. Best of all, since she absolutely loved the feeling of being on the water, she found herself rowing almost every other day. It didn't feel like exercise. Rather, it was feeding her soul and making her body feel good as a side bonus.

This is an excellent example of someone who made the effort to get to know herself and honor where she was in the present moment. You can do the same. Instead of cursing those two left feet, look at the situation differently. Think of it as a fun challenge to find something that completely works for you. You may be pleasantly surprised as you explore these new worlds.

I was recently introduced to the Japanese concept of kintsugi—the art of putting broken pottery pieces back together using a lacquer mixed with gold powder. This is built upon the idea of embracing flaws and imperfections in order to create an even stronger, more unique, and beautiful piece of art. Likewise, I encourage you to appreciate and own your flaws and imperfections. They have made you uniquely *you*. Striving for an unrealistic ideal life would not only be exhausting, but also wouldn't be authentic. It's better to accept and celebrate the whole *you* before beginning your journey.

Flaws and imperfections are your badge of courage and strength, a concrete reminder of a time where you had to overcome an obstacle. Instead of hiding them or holding any shame, celebrate those scars—whether physical or emotional—and use them to become uniquely better. We've all come from our own challenges and walks of life, which makes each of us uniquely different. In the process of bettering yourself while honoring your history, flaws, and imperfections, you will create an even more resilient and beautiful being. Reframing your hard times will remind you that you're not a victim of circumstance. You have control over the outcome of your stories. You get to choose how you live your life at any time. You'd never know the joys and brilliance of life without the full experience of the tough times as well. There has to be some level of hardship in order to appreciate your life and what you have.

So many of my clients start their wellness journey with their head full of shame and criticism. They focus on what's wrong versus what's right. By letting the negativity overtake you, any results you get will be short term. If you constantly feel like you're walking that high wire of perfection and worrying about stepping slightly off the path, what quality of life will you be leading? You've got to stop focusing on the negative and start being kind to yourself.

Look in the mirror and appreciate those flaws and imperfections as lessons to help guide your way forward. They are opportunities to learn more about yourself, to realize what worked and what didn't. Let these lessons empower you to tap into your inner strengths. Overcome what doesn't work for you and focus on the potential that does. We all know that our inner strength is so much more powerful than longer legs, a flat belly, or the ability to fit into the jeans you wore in high school.

RECOGNIZE AND USE YOUR STRENGTHS

It is so important to use your strengths and leverage your skills, especially when it comes to meeting your goals (and I don't just mean your wellness goals). One of the main concepts of positive psychology is discovering your signature strengths. These are the most prominent aspects that matter most to you. They're central to your personal identity. When you use these, it will feel natural and effortless. You will be happy, in balance, and ready to take on more challenges.

There's a nonprofit organization called the VIA Institute on Character that is dedicated to sharing the science of character strengths with the world. They've created surveys that help you find the most positive parts of your personality that impact how you think, feel, and behave. Over fifty-five scientists have worked to identify twenty-four character strengths that all human beings have the capacity to express. These scientists have learned how to specifically measure these character strengths in individuals. Each character strength falls under six broad virtue categories, which are universal across cultures and nations. Here's the breakdown:

CHARACTER STRENGTHS

1. **Wisdom and Knowledge**

    - Creativity (originality; ingenuity)
    - Curiosity (interest; openness to experiences)
    - Judgment (critical thinking)
    - Love of Learning (mastering new skills and topics; adding to knowledge)
    - Perspective (big-picture view)

2. **Courage and Valor**

    - Bravery (not shrinking from fear; speaking up for what's right)

- Perseverance (persistence)
- Honesty (authenticity; integrity)
- Zest (vitality; vigor)

3. **Humanity**

- Love (loving others and being loved; valuing close relationships with others)
- Kindness (generosity; compassion)
- Social Intelligence (emotional intelligence)

4. **Justice**

- Teamwork (citizenship; loyalty)
- Fairness (just; unbiased)
- Leadership (organization; motivator)

5. **Temperance**

- Forgiveness (mercy; accepting of others' shortcomings)
- Humility (modesty)
- Prudence (cautious; not taking undue risks)

- Self-Regulation (self-control; disciplined)

6. **Transcendence**

- Appreciation of Beauty/Excellence (awe; wonder)
- Gratitude (thankfulness)
- Hope (optimism; future orientation)
- Humor (playfulness; levity)
- Spirituality (faith; purpose; meaning)

One of my clients was recently diagnosed with an autoimmune condition. Understandably, there was some panic along with the stark realization that she needed to make big life changes in order to live a happy and healthy life. I had her take the VIA survey and we found that some of her top signature strengths were the love of learning, creativity, and courage. Using this knowledge, she was able to frame her condition as an opportunity to learn more about what was happening within her body. She used her creativity to come up with new recipes that would fall within her new eating plan. Best of all, she used her courage to face the new challenges that came with this condition. She had successfully adapted her lifestyle to meet her present condition and is still thriving to this day as a result.

She told me that, at first, she was angry and confused about her diagnosis. "I knew I had to make some major changes and I felt cheated. By using my character strengths, I was able to overcome this new challenge. It wasn't hard at all. It sounds really weird, but it felt natural once I understood everything." What better reason than this client's story to motivate you to understand your own character strengths?

I highly recommend that you take the VIA Survey of Character Strengths for yourself. Your signature strengths are the core of your identity. They should feel authentic and come naturally, and you should feel energized when you use them. Studies show that people have a high level of well-being when using their signature strengths regularly.

Psst. . . The VIA survey is free! All you have to do is register. The link is www.viacharacter.org/survey, and I recommend taking this survey again periodically. I have found that my own character strengths change over time because I'm continually evolving.

UNDERSTAND HOW YOU WORK

I ask my clients to fill out a questionnaire before we work together. The questions are a catalyst to understanding your own style and how you like to approach challenges.

GETTING TO KNOW YOURSELF

1. **What are you most proud of in your life so far?**

   This will give you an idea of what you feel you're capable of (there's that self-efficacy again). It will also take you down Memory Lane and remind yourself what you've accomplished, which will increase your confidence.

2. **What's important to you?**

   This will help you determine and set your priorities.

3. **What is the biggest thing you've had to overcome? What made it difficult? What did you learn from the experience?**

   This will help you remember that you've met challenges and overcame them in the past. It will also remind you what strengths and skills worked toward your success.

4. **How do you approach challenges?**

   This will help you understand your unique style and approach. While you plan your journey, you want to keep this question in mind and leverage your strengths and approaches to your advantage.

5. **Are you mostly past-, present-, or future-oriented?**

> This is sort of a trick question. If you find yourself to be past- or future-oriented, it may set up some obstacles. You may find yourself stuck in the past ("Last time I gained ten pounds, I lost it easily without exercise by simply portioning my meals."). While something may have worked in your twenties, it's likely different now. Alternatively, if you're caught up in the future ("I'll start dating when I lose ten pounds."), you'll constantly be holding yourself back from opportunities. If you don't lose the weight, does this mean you won't be able to date? Instead, I encourage you to focus on the present moment, this focus will help you see clearly, understand what resources you have, and know how to apply them.

As you read over these questions, are you beginning to assess where you're starting from? Note that there is absolutely no judgment here—nothing is good or bad, it just *is*. Don't spend any more time or energy worried about whether you have what it takes (you do!). Focus on becoming aware of how you work. What works for one person doesn't necessarily work for another. Fortunately, there are millions of ways to get to a single destination, and you get to choose the path that works best for you. Avoid allowing frustration and discouragement to seep in by recognizing what doesn't fit with who you are or how you work. Try an alternate program or method until you find one that does.

Take the time to develop your very own customized approach and strategy that will work for you. Get inspired by others and adopt and adapt different parts of various approaches. Honor yourself and celebrate your strengths, cultivate what you feel you're lacking, and understand that you're on a road trip! Things may change as you continue down the road to wellness, and that's okay. You are moving toward a healthier lifestyle, and that's the ultimate goal—it doesn't matter *how* you get there. Along the way, you'll discover who you really are and what elements help you find success. Revel in your uniqueness and recalibrate the behavior that you'd like to work toward.

Your endgame is to find the balance between your optimum health and living your life to the fullest. Enjoy that special day with good food and wine and return, with joy, to your regular days of healthy food. Use this road trip to celebrate your character and strengths while honoring your style and perspective. And if you find that this present path doesn't work or serve you the way it did in the past, make the choice to find a new path. Use what you already have and evolve into the person you know you can be.

SELF-ASSESSMENT

When I meet new clients, one of the first things I like to do with them is look at the Wellness Wheel. This is a great way to discover and prioritize which areas of your life need attention. How else will you know where you want to travel to if you don't know where you are starting from?

THE WELLNESS WHEEL

There are many life and wellness assessments online, and you can choose to do any one of them (type "free wellness life assessment tools" in your search engine). Or because this book is so interesting and you can't tear yourself away from it, let's create your own Wellness Wheel. Take a piece of paper and draw a big circle (it doesn't have to be perfect). Divide it into eight sections and label each one as shown below.

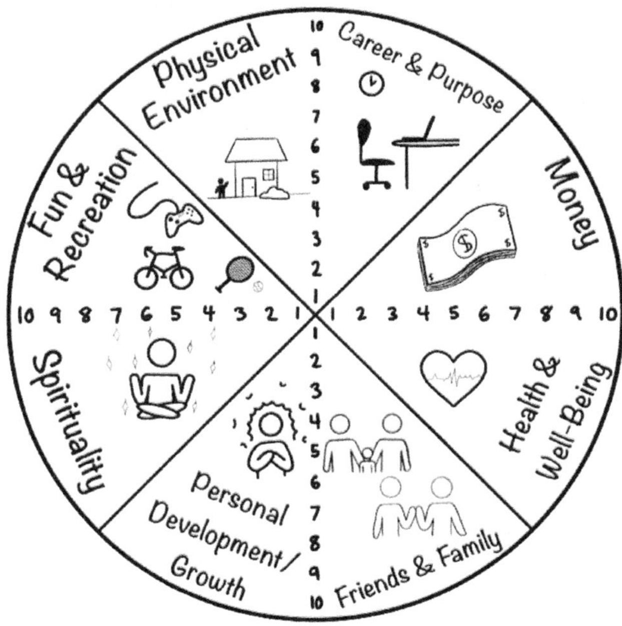

Read through the following questions and give each section a value on a scale of one to ten, with one being, "I need to work on this STAT," and ten being, "I've got this. I should be teaching other people how to do it!" Be brutally honest when answering these questions. This will adequately represent your satisfaction with each section of your life.

PHYSICAL ENVIRONMENT

1. How do you feel about where you live?

2. Does your home give or take energy?

3. Is your home peaceful or chaotic? Can you relax or are you constantly on edge?

4. Are you comfortable letting outsiders see where you live? Do you have pride in your home and neighborhood?

5. Do you feel safe and secure?

CAREER/PURPOSE

1. How satisfied are you with your purpose? Is it stimulating, rewarding, and reflective of your values?

2. Do you feel like you're making a difference?

3. Are you using your talents and passions to support others?

4. How do you feel on the evening before your work week begins? Are you excited or depressed?

5. What do you do on a weekly basis that makes you feel like you're positively impacting the world?

MONEY

1. Are you living within your means and responsible for your financial decisions?
2. Are your spending and saving habits reflecting your values and beliefs?
3. Are you planning for periods in your life when you might not have an active income?
4. Are you paying bills on time and managing credit positively?
5. Are you balancing present-day spending with saving for the future?

HEALTH AND WELL-BEING

1. How do you feel about yourself?
2. How often do you move throughout the day?
3. What is your typical mood during an average day?
4. How much energy do you have?

5. Are you eating well? Do you feel good after you eat?

6. How are you sleeping? Are you refreshed when you wake up?

7. Are you taking care of your health with regular medical and dental checkups? Are you following your doctor's recommendations?

8. Do you have or are you at risk for any chronic ailments?

FAMILY AND FRIENDS

1. Are you satisfied with your relationships?

2. Are you able to resolve conflicts in all areas of your life?

3. Are you satisfied with your social interactions with others?

4. Can you set and respect your own and other people's boundaries?

5. How aware are you of the feelings of others? Can you respond appropriately?

6. Do you have a sense of belonging within a group or an organization?

7. Are you spending quality time with your loved ones? How connected do you feel to them?

PERSONAL DEVELOPMENT/GROWTH

1. Do you make time for personal growth?
2. Do you have a sense of control in your life?
3. How are you able to adapt to change?
4. What coping mechanism do you use? Are you able to comfort or console yourself when you're troubled?
5. Do you feel responsible for your feelings and how you express them?
6. Are you confident and open to new challenges?
7. Are you disciplined and accountable?

SPIRITUALITY

1. Do you have a sense of meaning and purpose in your life?
2. Do you have a general sense of serenity and contentment?
3. Are you satisfied with your principles, ethics, and morals? Do they provide guidance for your life?
4. Are you able to trust others and have the ability to forgive others and yourself?

5. Do you take specific time to contemplate and explore your beliefs and spirituality?

FUN AND RECREATION

1. Do you have activities that bring you joy and give you something to look forward to?
2. How satisfied are you with your current work/life balance?
3. Do you have enough "me" time?
4. Is there anything that you'd like to try, learn, or do that you haven't done yet?

My Wellness Wheel changes every month when I do this exercise to check in with myself. Since this is YOUR wheel, you also can create your own customized categories that are closer to your values and priorities.

It's important that you withhold judgment. The short spokes only illustrate that you've paid less attention to those areas, not that you are failing. Use this information to see where you can grow and improve. Don't forget to take into account what's happening in your life at the time or if you're feeling overwhelmed or stressed. For example, when I'm working under deadlines, my career has a stronger focus for a time. But when I'm on vacation, fun and recreation take priority. And that's okay!

Everything in your life is connected. For example, if you lack health, most of the other areas in your life will suffer such as your finances, relationships, environment, and fun. Personally, I believe your purpose is pretty high in importance too. If you don't know or understand your purpose, it can be challenging to find the motivation to change the other areas in your life.

The goal of the Wellness Wheel exercise is to make sure that your life is balanced. It's very natural to give too much attention to one or two areas, and not enough to others. If we're not aware of what's going on in all the areas of our lives, we may feel unsettled and incomplete without understanding why.

SETTING YOUR VISION

Now that you have an idea of what areas of your life could use a little help, it's time for the fun part—setting your vision. Articulating and developing a compelling version of your future self will make it easier for you to determine the person you want to be.

Although it's good to know what you don't want, focusing on what you *do* want can be more motivational and uplifting. Make sure your vision is detailed and personalized to *your* needs and desires. If your vision is driven by outside forces or the need for validation (based on what others want from you), it won't be deeply rooted enough to motivate you and keep you on track. Prioritizing *your* feelings will help you stay true to yourself and make this road trip more authentic, enjoyable, and successful.

Here's a five- to ten-minute exercise that can help you visualize your future-self. Get some paper and a pen to jot down your notes as you go.

SETTING YOUR VISION

Find a quiet place where you won't be disturbed. Start by taking a couple of slow, deep breaths to quiet your mind. As you feel yourself settling into a state of calmness, imagine a place where you feel comfortable, peaceful, strong, and confident.

1. **What does this place look like? How do you feel when you're there?**

   Take the time to describe this place in detail. How does this place feel to you? What is making you relaxed and comfortable?

2. **Picture yourself six months, one year, and five years from now.**

   How do you feel physically? How do you look physically? What are you wearing? How does your body move? Take the time to notice any other changes from where you are right now.

3. **Imagine what you did to become your future-self.**

   What did you have to do to get there? What activities are you doing as your future-self? What does it feel like? What are you doing differently? Who's around you?

You should now have a pretty good idea of how you want your future-self to be. Test your future-self with the following questions. I recommend that you write your visions in present tense as if they were already happening. Also, write them in your voice as if you were talking to a dear friend (we're more likely to be supportive and encouraging to others than ourselves).

1. **Value** – Is your future-self a compelling statement of who you are now? Does your future-self incorporate behaviors you want to do consistently?

2. **Thrive** – What makes you thrive? When are you most alive?

3. **Strengths** – What's working? What are you doing to support your well-being? What part of your life do you feel best about?

4. **Importance** – What is the most important thing to you? What element of your well-being do you want to improve?

5. **Motivation** – What will be the benefits of making these changes? What is the driving force behind your vision?

VISION BOARD

Craft your vision further by creating a vision board. These tools are great because they can continually remind you of what your future-self will be. I look at my vision board every day to remind myself what I'm working toward and to maintain my motivation. When I uncover a potential opportunity, I always do a quick check on my vision board to make sure that the opportunity aligns with my endgame. If it doesn't, it could be distracting you from your ultimate goals.

Some people are really creative, but even if you're not (I'm in this category), I've found that the following vision board exercise has worked wonderfully for me. You can create your vision board in any way that you want, but it's REALLY important to understand what you're working toward. Once you put all the information together, your vision board will help you understand and reach your goal.

Ready to be honest with yourself and discover your vision? The following questions will help you figure out what you want most out of your life. Use just one or two words to answer them on both a personal and a professional level.

1. **The Why** – What are the most important factors in your life?

2. **Non-Negotiables** – What are your non-negotiables? What can't be ignored or pushed aside?

3. **I Want** – What do you want more of in your life?

4. **Cultivate** – What qualities do you want to cultivate in yourself? Who do you want to become this year?

5. **Feeling** – How do you want to feel at the end of next year?

6. **Need More Of**– What's missing or needs to be included so that you can reach the rest of your goals?

Once you've answered all of the questions, you can cut them out and place them on a poster board where you can see it every day. I chose instead to create a PowerPoint so I could have it with me in digital format everywhere I go. I look at

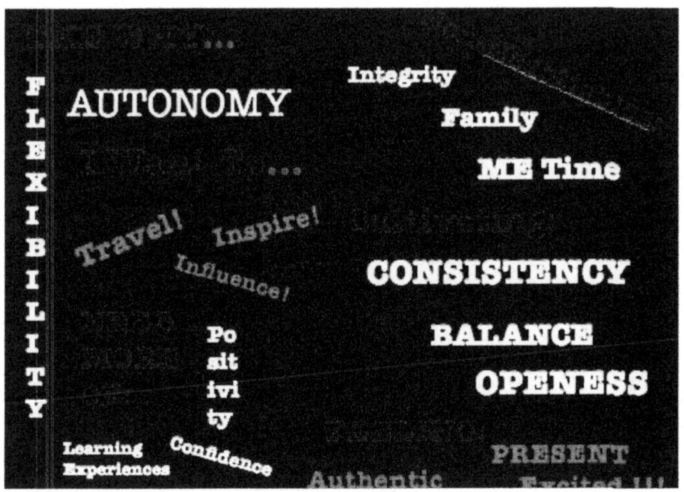

it each morning to keep myself on track, and also when I feel lost or distracted.

By now, you should have your vision solidified. You should have a clear view of what you would like in your life and which areas should be prioritized or improved upon. You should also understand where you're starting from—who you are, your strengths, and your preferred style.

All of this information will help you move forward, especially when times get rough and you run into obstacles. Through these exercises, you've given life to your vision. You know how you want to feel and what aligns with your purpose and your values. With a strong vision, you'll be able to move those obstacles out of your way and progress toward living your vision!

DESTINATIONS

"Once a year, go somewhere you've never been before."
– The Dalai Lama
2022

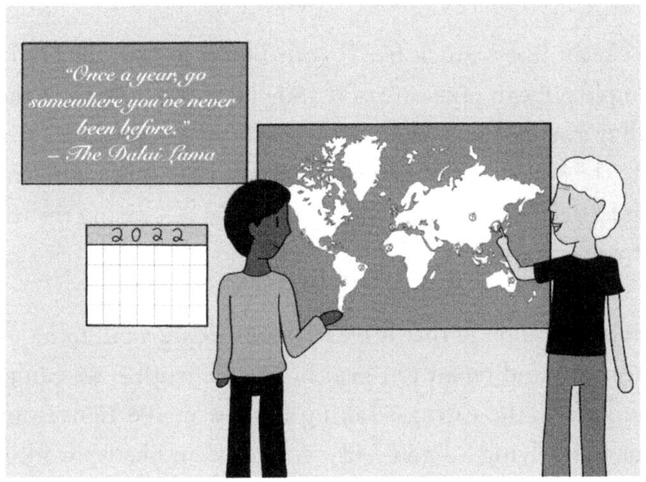

Now we get to the fun part—planning your itinerary! This is a great opportunity to visit areas that you may be curious about but have never experienced. As you remember, we are defining destinations as the areas that we want to visit or explore in our lives, the lifestyle habits and trouble spots that we want to adopt or change. Experience and exposure in these areas will help us obtain the vision that we worked on earlier.

Admittedly, there are an infinite number of destinations that exist, and I definitely don't want to overwhelm you. So, for this road trip that we journey on together, let's limit the choices within the functional medicine world. Once you get the hang of this, the world is your oyster. You will be able to explore many more destinations and even create a destination customized to your needs and vision!

FUNCTIONAL MEDICINE

We'd all like a quick fix. If your blood pressure is high, a simple pill can take care of it and you won't have to change what you eat or drink. You could continue to live your life the way you want. It's effortless to be in denial or not understand that this very lifestyle could be causing the root of your problems.

I wish I could say that it *is* as easy as taking a pill to fix our problems and repair our health, but the truth is we can get worse from these drugs. Taking all these medications is similar to applying a Band-Aid—it may seem like it's working at first because you've covered it up. But underneath, the wound is festering, and other problems are arising. We can become more stressed, feel even worse than we did to begin with, and continue to soothe ourselves with our unhealthy lifestyle (likely creating more problems). Not only that, but the simple pill that was supposed to take care of our blood pressure now puts us at risk for yet another chronic disease and can lose its effectiveness as your body adjusts to it.

I'm beginning to observe more and more people who don't want to live life this way, and bravo to them! If we can learn to switch our focus from a quick fix to a real fix, we could heal in more ways than expected. As time moves forward, our eyes are opening to this fact. We're slowly becoming more invested in our health and taking accountability for how we can live healthier lives without dependence on that quick fix that doesn't truly fix anything after all. Instead of a Band-Aid, let's find the root of the problem and repair it.

Functional medicine differs from conventional Western medicine in this manner by directly addressing the restoration of health. Instead of simply treating the symptoms with drugs, the goal is to find out what's causing the problem in the first place and figure out how to let your body do what it does best—heal itself. By focusing on finding the root causes among the symptoms and diagnoses, functional medicine seeks to eliminate the disease itself.

This makes total sense, right? Wouldn't it be better to remove the root cause of the symptom than to take a prescription that can only treat a specific symptom? The functional medicine approach supports this holistic line of thinking, and more and more physicians and their patients are favoring this approach when faced with chronic health issues. Personally, I believe (and hope) that functional medicine will be the future approach to healthcare. It's amazing how quickly someone can restore their health with consistency and focus. It's not easy, but I truly believe it's worth the extra effort. Can you imagine how good it will be when you don't have to deal with pain or health issues over and over again? Repairing the issue from the roots will *heal* your body!

As a holistic approach to health, functional medicine looks at health as a whole. You're not just focusing on what you eat but also how often you move, how well you sleep, how you manage your stress, and how connected you feel to others. All these areas play a big part in how you feel at the end of the day.

To clarify, functional medicine does not do away with Western medicine. Instead, it aims to work alongside it and offer a flexible perspective on treatment approaches. As I'm sure you'll agree, we are not all alike. Our genes are different, our bodies are different, and our desires are different. What works for each individual is rarely the same. Therefore, you need a flexible customized solution to help what's ailing you. That may include a pill with your daily exercise and healthier diet, or it may not.

There are some things we all do have in common. For example, there are seven interrelated physiological processes that tell us how our body functions—digestion and assimilation, detoxification, defense and repair, cellular communication, cellular transportation, energy, and structure. Functional medicine states that any breakdown or difficulty within these seven systems will lead to health issues and, eventually, chronic illness. If there's an imbalance in one or more of these core processes, the altered function is likely to cause an ailment. Our behaviors and actions play a key role in our genetic function. Every component in our body communicates to each other, and when one is down, the rest will be impacted. Your lifestyle plays a big role in functional medicine. In fact, your lifestyle can be the "medicine" that helps you get better.

Personalized treatments and preventive actions are the two elements that will successfully bring your core physiological processes back into balance. However, this can't be accomplished unless the patient is committed to making those lifestyle changes. Changing your lifestyle will cost far less than medications and will play a long-term role in getting you back to the healthy person you want to be. By changing the environment, you can bring these components back into balance and let these core processes function the way they're supposed to.

There are five functional medicine lifestyle factors (FMLF) that make up the "environment" that surrounds your genes. These will be our destinations on our wellness journeys.

DESTINATIONS

1. Nutrition and Hydration
2. Mobility, Movement, and Exercise
3. Sleep and Relaxation
4. Stress Management
5. Connection

After completing the Wellness Wheel exercise, you probably have some idea of the areas that you'd like to work on and explore. There's a wonderful way you can integrate this information with the lifestyle factors above.

As an example, let's say the three sections that ranked the lowest on your Wellness Wheel were health and well-being, career and purpose, and friends and family. How does the FMLF impact these areas?

Health and Well-Being – How do you feel physically? Are you ready for your day with good nutrition and rest? Can you enjoy physical activity? Can you rest easily, or do you always feel like you need to be productive? Can you turn your thoughts off at night? Do you feel that your lack of energy keeps you from connecting with others?

Career and Purpose – Do you have enough energy and mobility to complete your work to your full potential? Do you start each day refreshed and ready to tackle all your professional challenges? Do you feel supported by your work group and your family?

Friends and Family – Relationships take energy. Are you nourishing yourself and getting enough rest to feel good? Are you mobile enough to go and enjoy time with the people close to you? Can you relax enough to be present and have a good time? Are you finding it easy to connect with your current friends and/or make new ones?

BREAKING IT INTO DAY TRIPS

Attaining an outcome that matches your vision requires actual behavioral changes. By exploring your larger goals (destinations) and breaking them into smaller goals (day trips or tours), you'll be able to discover and try different actions and approaches to not only make those changes, but also get them to stick! Your day trips will allow you to spend time exploring and applying what you learn to your life. You'll be exposed to things like trying different foods, setting a nighttime routine that will help you sleep better, and learning to meditate to reduce your stress. The possibilities are endless, not to mention the crossover benefits!

If you're working on nutrition and hydration, you might take a "vegetable tour" to open yourself up to the possibility of eating more vegetables. You're going to learn what new dishes to try and decide how often and how many vegetables you'll eat. You might also consider investing in a shiny new water bottle to help ensure that you remember to drink enough water. While working on nutrition and hydration, you may find yourself having increased energy as a bonus benefit.

If you're exploring the mobility, movement, and exercise destination, you want to find a good exercise program that you actually enjoy. Maybe you'll go on two tours and try both yoga and dance. Before the tours, you're going to do the research to understand the benefits. Then, while on the tours, you'll likely need to try different classes to figure out what you like and what you'll stick with for the long haul.

While working on this destination, you may also build some new connections in your classes and find that you're sleeping better at night.

While visiting the stress management destination, establishing a wind-down routine could help you sleep better so you can take on your stressors with a rested body. Taking a meditation tour could help you let go of your stressors so, rather than feeling like you're going to snap, you can handle whatever happens. Along the way, you may start to realize that you eat when you're overwhelmed and stressed, and maybe you feel inspired to replace unhealthy snacks with healthier alternatives.

The connection destination could guide you to new connections or lead you to join new support groups that will help you stick to your healthier eating plan. In addition, building connections will help you feel supported, validated, cared for, and fulfilled. Feeling happier and more fulfilled will lead you to continue making those healthy choices at mealtimes, and maybe you even join an exercise class with one of your new connections.

I hope you can see how making changes to your lifestyle might be fun and reap multiple benefits. You are on an adventure to wellness! You're exposing yourself to things that are new and exciting, building new connections, and feeling refreshed and able to handle whatever comes your way. You'll always be able to revisit places that you love and get to know them even better. Are you getting excited about your road trip?

Let's take a closer look into your destination options and how the FMLF fit in. We'll also explore some possible day tour ideas you could take.

NUTRITION AND HYDRATION

When someone complains about being tired or feeling run down, one of my first questions is, "What have you been eating?" Often, we don't connect our diet to the rest of our well-being. You may be portioning well, but not eating the right foods. Our body has to work harder to process the toxins found in certain foods and the environment. If we aren't feeding our bodies with the nutrition it needs to function properly, it's no wonder that our body doesn't function properly! It's easier to get the job done well if you have the proper tools.

More than half of our immune system resides in our digestive tract. Unfortunately, much of the foods that we consume are overly refined and processed, filled with chemicals and hormones, and tax our digestive tracts and detoxification systems. When alien substances like processed foods, inflammatory fats, gluten, and excess sugar are detected, our defense system attacks the invaders. In an effort to protect our bodies from harm, our immune system goes into fire/inflammation mode. If your body has been doing this for much of your life, you will find that you're having problems with your health and wellness, likely caused by your defense system being overwhelmed.

As we get older, we tend to generate more food allergies and sensitivities. Current research shows that one out of ten adults has or will develop a food allergy. Certain foods such as dairy, nuts, eggs, and wheat can trigger uncomfortable reactions such as swelling and inflammation. We can also develop food intolerances. This happens when we're not allergic to the actual food, but we have trouble digesting it. The most common intolerances are gluten and lactose (found in most dairy foods), and the best recommendation is to limit or eliminate these foods altogether from your diet.

Lack of proper hydration can also affect how you feel. Most of the time when we feel hungry, we are actually just thirsty. In a survival situation, the top priority is always to find water, then food. Sixty percent of our body is water. That's more than half! It makes sense, then, that when we are dehydrated, our bodies don't function as well and can even lead us into health complications.

Drinking water replenishes important minerals like potassium, magnesium, and sodium. Water also aids your body in distributing these important chemicals to your organs, tissues, and other bodily systems, which all require water to function properly. When your body can function as designed, you're able to maintain a healthy blood pressure, eliminate waste from your cells, and regulate your body temperature. Staying hydrated helps to facilitate all the bodily functions needed to keep you feeling good and healthy.

SHOULD YOU ADD THE NUTRITION AND HYDRATION DESTINATION TO YOUR ITINERARY?

- How do you feel after you eat?
- Do you have enough energy to do the things you enjoy? Do you accomplish the goals you set for your day?
- How alert and productive are you? Are there any times that you feel better or worse than other times?
- Are you eating to nourish your body, or are you eating to soothe your feelings?

POSSIBLE DAY TRIPS FOR THE NUTRITION AND HYDRATION DESTINATION:

- Explore, discover, and make the connection of how food impacts the way you feel. Consider keeping a journal where you can write brief notes about what you ate, note the time, and follow up with how you felt afterward.
- Using the knowledge gained from your food journal, replace the foods that don't make you feel good with foods that make you feel great.
- Improve your digestion by focusing on mindful eating.

- Understand and choose the best eating plan for you. Find one that allows you to consistently stick with it. You want to find foods that you enjoy and also help you feel your best. Your goal is to feel satisfied, happy, and good about yourself!

MOBILITY, MOVEMENT, AND EXERCISE

When I was in my thirties, I still jumped out of bed every day for my early morning run. Fast forward to my fifties and you'll find me slowly waking my body each morning. I feel like a relative of the rusty Tin Man. It's a cruel twist of nature that we move less as we grow older. The lack of movement can create low-grade inflammation throughout your body. It's the age-old adage (pun intended) of "use it or lose it." Bottom line, we *need* to move in order to be healthy.

I would say that the number one reason why people exercise is to control their weight, but it's not *just* about the weight. Exercise helps you fight chronic diseases as well as manage mental anxiety. Moving can also improve your mood—it's all about the endorphins that are released when you do something that makes you feel good. As a side benefit, you'll also feel better about your appearance and increase your self-confidence. When I'm lethargic, I find that moving increases my energy! Weird, but true. It also puts your cardiovascular system to use, improves your muscle strength, and builds endurance. In addition, regular physical activity can help you fall asleep faster, deeper, and better—just be sure to not be too active right before bedtime. And these are just a few benefits to exercise!

Even with all of these benefits, this is often the most challenging habit to adapt to. Many of my clients will do great in the first couple of months, but then life gets busy, and exercise is put on the back burner.

Need some tips to help you stick to this essential healthy habit? Understand that you not only need to make time in your schedule, but also adopt the mindset that will help you commit and sustain a regular exercise routine. Accountability is the most effective element in making sure you stick to your exercise. The support of a loved one, workout buddy, or a group with common goals will help you keep it up, especially at the beginning when you're still establishing the habit. Also be sure to begin with baby steps. Instead of committing to a yoga class every day, start with just two or three days a week. Jumping in full force can overwhelm you and cause you to quit but completing small goals will increase your confidence and connect you with the benefits without completely overhauling your life.

It's also important to pick an activity that you will enjoy. Many of my clients commit to going to the gym every other day and then tell me that they hate going to the gym. I can almost guarantee that if you are forcing yourself to do something that you hate, you will not be doing it in the future. Instead, think of something that brings you joy. It could be going outside for a walk, hitting a ball to release your frustrations, putting on great dance music and moving like no one is watching (this is my jam!). If you don't know what to choose, explore the exercise programs out there that can make it fun, like kickboxing, tai chi, dance workouts, or yoga. Whatever you choose, you need to associate positive emotions with the activity so your unconscious mind will steer you to want to do it more often. You don't have to choose just one option either. You can mix your exercise program up! As we age, we want to make sure that we have a healthy balance of endurance, strength, and stretching. If you get bored easily, make sure that you alternate different workouts to avoid getting into a rut while also working your body from several different angles.

SHOULD YOU ADD THE MOBILITY, MOVEMENT, AND EXERCISE DESTINATION TO YOUR ITINERARY?

- How do you feel about exercise? Do you have negative or positive feelings? What can you do to change them to be more positive?

- How do you feel after exercising versus before exercising? Do you notice a difference in your mood, muscles, and mind?

- What does your body call out for? Do you feel nervous energy? Exhausted? Strong? Many times, it helps to just listen to your body and choose a cardio, strength, or restorative type of exercise that works for you.

POSSIBLE DAY TRIPS FOR THE MOBILITY, MOVEMENT, AND EXERCISE DESTINATION:

- Explore, discover, and make the connection of how movement impacts the way you feel. Keep an exercise journal and take notes both before and after your workout or activity.

- Find activities that you really enjoy and don't dread performing.

- Find workout buddies (mine are my three dogs) to enjoy your workout with.

- Find accountability partners and systems to help you stick to your exercise plan that you designed for yourself.

SLEEP AND RELAXATION

"I'll sleep when I'm dead."

How many times have we heard this phrase, or even said it ourselves? Why is sleep so undervalued in our society? As I'm sure we've all experienced at one time or another, a good night's sleep can make or break your day.

Some benefits to being well-rested are the ability to resist infections and promote a healthier immune system, repair and restore our bodies in addition to detoxification, promote emotional well-being as well as give the brain time to restore itself by forming new pathways, and prevent weight gain and improve appetite regulation.

"Okay, okay. . . I get the benefits of sleep, but I'm horrible at sleeping. There's too much to do and not enough time."

This is something I hear from my clients when we talk about sleep. I know this all too well because I'm formerly one of the worst sleepers ever. I stayed up way too late and got up way too early to get everything checked off my to-do list. Ironically, my days weren't as productive as they could've been. Also due to those eighteen-hour days, I carried an extra ten pounds on my exhausted body.

Experts all around agree that sleep can be improved through learning and practicing better sleep hygiene. This means no more boot camp classes right before we go to bed and turn off your screens at least two hours before you need to sleep. A regular night routine does wonders. I use a meditation exercise when the lights go off to get my brain to power down.

SHOULD YOU ADD THE SLEEP AND RELAXATION DESTINATION TO YOUR ITINERARY?

- Is lack of sleep disrupting your life?
- What is the source of your sleep difficulty?

- What habits do you have that are preventing you from getting a good night's sleep?

- Are you dependent on unhealthy substances to help you sleep?

- How is your overall well-being?

POSSIBLE DAY TRIPS FOR THE SLEEP AND RELAXATION DESTINATION:

- Understand the importance of sleep and how it impacts your body. Being well-rested can affect all the other areas of your life. Lack of proper rest can impact your efficiency, immune system, and even your weight. Consider keeping a sleep journal where you note what you did in the hour or two before sleep, log how many hours of sleep you get, and how you feel in the morning.

- Make improvements to your sleep hygiene by maintaining a consistent sleep schedule. Shut off electronics at least two hours before you need to sleep and instead, allow yourself time to relax at the end of the day. Calm your nervous system down by reading, meditating, or doing restorative yoga.

- Set yourself up for quality sleep. Consider investing in blackout curtains, a sleep mask, or a white noise machine. You might also consider using a fitness tracker to measure the quality of your sleep and learn how you could improve it. Ensure you don't partake in any consumption that could disrupt your sleep, such as a late coffee, alcoholic drink, or sugar.

STRESS MANAGEMENT

Everyone has stress. It's an unfortunate and inevitable occurrence in our lives. But contrary to what some people believe, stress can be a good thing—in moderation. Stress is used by our bodies as a survival tactic. Acute stress (a clear beginning and end point) can help us stay motivated, work toward goals, and feel good about our lives.

Think about joining a new class or meeting a new person. This may bring you a little stress, but it's also something that you're excited about. This is known as eustress, the beneficial stress that brings on optimal performance. Working and exploring outside of your comfort zone is healthy. It challenges you to grow emotionally, psychologically, and physically. Exploring new things is inherently stressful because we don't know what will happen or how it will turn out. Deciding to take your road trip to wellness is a great example of eustress! It should be a little scary, but also very exciting. You'll endure feelings and situations that will be foreign to you. For many, it will be an eye-opening experience that will help you learn more about yourself.

The challenge is to make sure that eustress doesn't become distress. Distress happens when we let the stress overwhelm us. Usually, this happens because our physiological, cognitive, and coping resources are inadequate for the challenges we're facing.

There are three ways an individual can respond to stressors.

PHYSIOLOGICAL

While everyone has the same basic stress physiology, there are differences within our individual responses that originate from our genetics, culture, and past experiences. By being aware of what makes you tick and what your reactions are, you can manage your stress successfully.

Your physiological reactivity involves your nervous system and your brain. Without getting too technical, we have two aspects to our nervous system—the sympathetic (SNS) and the parasympathetic (PNS). The first triggers our "fight or flight" instinct, and the latter is "rest and digest."

When there's a stressor that's determined to be a threat, our nerves stimulate different organs in our body. Our heart rate increases, and our adrenals are activated as our body gets ready to "fight or take flight." Cortisol increases our blood sugar, suppresses our immune system, and aids in the metabolism of fat, protein, and carbohydrates. These processes help prepare our bodies to fight stressors.

When the stress is eliminated, our nervous system downshifts into the "rest and digest" mode. This phase allows our nervous system to return us back to the balanced body, restoring it to the state of calm, and allows the body to relax, rejuvenate, and repair. Acute stress is inevitable and normal. What's not normal is to be in constant chronic stress—when your "fight or flight" system is working overtime.

Symptoms of chronic stress include muscle tension, pain, headaches, IBS, gas, bloating, skin reactions, respiratory issues, inflammation, sleep disturbances, loss of focus, poor memory, anxiety and depression, inability to maintain good relationships, poor job performance, and poor sense of self. These are just a handful of the possible symptoms, and as you can see, chronic stress can impact your physical, mental, and emotional abilities. Chronic stress occurs when we continually think and relive a negative event over and over, forcing ourselves to remain in a state of high distress.

COGNITIVE-EMOTIONAL APPRAISAL

Do you ever wonder why some people are continually stressed, and others don't seem to have a care in the world? Perception plays a big part in how we respond to stress. How you appraise a situation will be key in determining whether each event will be a stressor for you.

We all have our own individual perceptions and responses because of our genetics, culture, and past experiences. The trick is to understand that these factors may be influencing you to believe something is a dangerous threat, when in reality, maybe it isn't. Interestingly enough, if you feel that you're empowered or in control of your life, you may experience less chronic stress due to the fact that you understand that you can change it.

COPING MECHANISMS

Think of your emotions as energy in motion, impacting your mood and state of mind. We all have different thresholds and sensitivities to emotional stimuli, but your coping mechanisms and the way you react to certain situations plays a big role in your stress. Both negative and positive emotions can be powerful and have a large impact on your day.

Negative emotions can prepare you to act quickly, which helped our ancestors survive predators and threats that came their way. Similarly, it can help you respond quickly when in moments of danger. However, continual negative thinking can also have detrimental effects. Constant anger, fear, and frustration will suppress your immune system and may wreak havoc on your life and relationships, create additional stress, and lead to chronic health issues. This is an uncomfortable and a miserable state to be in.

You need to find a balance between the negative and the positive. Understand that the negative feelings are beneficial because they send you the message that something needs to change. But you can also use positive emotions to help you solve the issue once you've taken yourself to a place of safety. Positive emotions can broaden and build long-lasting personal resources. You can undo the lingering effects of the negative emotions ("Thank you for the warning, now please go away!") and generate resiliency in confronting those threats or stressors. You can use these emotions to invite more flexible thinking as well as request social support. Your body reacts well in a state of balance by enhancing your immune system and functions.

The good news is that you can become better at living with stress by embracing it and learning how to manage it when it comes your way. Adding the stress management destination to your itinerary will serve you in most anything that you strive for. It will help you understand the triggers that cause you stress and learn how to reframe and reinterpret this information to discover new management techniques that will greatly enrich your life.

SHOULD YOU ADD THE STRESS MANAGEMENT DESTINATION TO YOUR ITINERARY?

- Can you shut off at the end of the day or are you constantly replaying things over and over, worrying about the outcome?

- Are you treating yourself with care (good diet, plenty of rest, and activities that bring you joy)?

- Are you sleeping well?

- How often are you irritated, worked up, or anxious? Can you quickly move out of that mode to find relaxation and feel ready to take on the next thing?

- Are you developing bad habits (too much alcohol, eating junk food, binge watching television) to help yourself cope with the way you're feeling?

POSSIBLE DAY TRIPS FOR THE STRESS MANAGEMENT DESTINATION:

- Take a deep dive into what's stressing you out. Is it a temporary issue that can be fixed and forgotten? Is it a pattern that you need to reframe? Is it a story that is no longer serving you? Can you let it go?

- Have you packed too much into your to-do list? Are you prioritizing the things that mean the most to you? What can you let go of or postpone until a later time? Is there anything you can delegate to another person in your family or at your job?

- Have you set the boundaries of what's right for you? Are you trying to please others, or have you stepped into a role that is not meant for you?

- Is there an issue that you don't want to face? If so, what is holding you back from resolving it?

- Do you know where you're going or where you want to go? If not, do you have any areas of interest that you can research to find out if those are right for you?

CONNECTION

It's very important in today's society to be independent and self-sufficient. I'm not sure where we lost our way, but ultimately, I believe that everyone needs to connect with at least one other person. Science supports this concept. Psychological research has shown that good levels of social connection lead to better health and wellness. People with low social connection are at a higher risk for chronic diseases as well as depression, stress, and anxiety. Your brain and nervous system are primed with the need to belong. When you have intimacy with other human beings, neurochemicals are delivered to your brain, and your heart becomes warm and full (hence the term heartwarming). We are physiologically wired to build connections.

Human interaction is not simply something we desire, but an essential *need* for our wellness. Connections help us understand what's going on around us; they make us feel supported and a part of something larger than ourselves. They provide a sense of safety, give meaning to our presence, and encourage us to be who we really are. Connections establish the experience of oneness—having shared experiences, relatable feelings, or similar ideas. Matthew Lieberman, author of *Social: Why Our Brains Are Wired to Connect*, writes, "Love and belonging might seem like a convenience we can live without, but our biology is built to thirst for connection because it is linked to our most basic survival needs." Our need to connect is as fundamental as our need for food and water. You need a supportive environment and praise to motivate you to keep moving forward.

So, why is it so challenging to build deep connections sometimes? It takes courage to show your true, authentic self. There's a major fear of rejection, which would confirm your worst fear that "there's something wrong with me." The internet and social media increase your ability to be whoever you want to be (although inauthentic) and, therefore, protect yourself from potential rejection. You can gloat, edit, filter, and only post the positive highlights of your life if you wanted to. You can tell whatever "story" you want, but it may not be an honest reflection of your reality. Likewise, you may be getting the "filtered" version of another person in this manner.

This breeches true connection. It keeps you from really getting to know another person. It's easy to confuse attention for connection, but you and I both know that it's not the same thing! Connection is more intentional and thoughtful and focuses on giving more than receiving. Connection doesn't mean trying to earn approval, awe, compliments, or superiority. I know this won't surprise you, but connection begins with yourself—you've got to connect with your true self before you can have a deep connection with others. Give yourself permission to be open, show up just as you are, and trust that you'll make authentic connections. Have confidence in yourself. You are important. You are enough. And there are others out there who will cherish the real you—you just have to find them.

SHOULD YOU ADD THE CONNECTION DESTINATION TO YOUR ITINERARY?

- How "present" are your close relationships? Are you sharing who you really are or just playing a role?
- Do you feel alone in this world even though you're surrounded by people?
- Do you feel supported within the group you spend the most time with?
- Are you satisfied with the quality of your relationships? What could make them better?
- Sit with just yourself for a moment. Do you even know yourself? Do you know your own opinions, dreams, and what makes you happy?

POSSIBLE DAY TRIPS FOR THE CONNECTION DESTINATION:

- Learn more about yourself and understand what makes you tick, what makes you happy, and what you're scared of. Try new things. Imagine a future you and what sort of job, friends, and hobbies you'd have.

- Learn your strengths and weaknesses. Who are you with when you are the best version of you? What do you need? What can you leave behind?

- Take accountability for your own feelings without projecting them on the people around you. Be secure with who you are and share your true self with those who care about you and want you to be content. They don't necessarily have to be the same as you, they just need to care for you.

- Learn how to create and establish mutually trusting relationships. Understand and achieve the fine balance of giving and receiving.

PRIORITIZING YOUR ITINERARY

ONE ROAD TRIP AT A TIME

By now, I hope some of the destinations have piqued your interest and are getting you excited to start your road trip. If you're like me, you've probably picked out more than one destination to incorporate into your future vision.

I strongly advise that you only take one journey at a time. You could try them all at once, but you would likely get stressed out and quit on yourself before those changes really had a chance to take root. Too many changes all at once are a lot to take on and when we feel overwhelmed from the start, any little distraction can offset your progress. With too many balls up in the air, it would be really tempting to just give up. It will be much more effective to have one focus (or destination) at a time so you can fully enjoy all that each destination has to offer and make changes that will last a lifetime.

Remember that the objective of your road trip is to be fluid and flexible. If you hit an obstacle or a delay, you can easily zag instead of zig and still find success and enjoyment. There are so many unexpected events and opportunities in life. If we're too strict with our itineraries, you may lose out on some chances to see and experience exciting things. Aim for a specific direction but know that it's okay if you have to stop or take a different path to reach your destination. Being flexible will help you make the most of your energy and resources, making your trip valuable all the way around.

STAGES OF BEHAVIORAL CHANGE

Changing our behaviors is quite a challenge, especially when our lives have heavy demands and stressors that can deplete the energy needed to make them. If it were easy, you probably wouldn't have picked up this book. You wouldn't be seeking help on your journey. Research has shown that the very action of changing yourself is a staged process where you transition from pre-contemplation (not thinking about it) to contemplation (preparing for action) to actual action.

When I was trying to cut sugar, part of me was resistant because I really didn't believe that this would enhance my life. Rather, I looked at it as incurring a loss. I love sweets. I didn't see any benefit to something being taken away from me. Not surprisingly, there were a lot of stops and starts on that journey.

For me, quitting cold turkey was detrimental for my mindset. What I needed to understand was that I never truly made up my mind to give up sweets. Taking away the sugar applied pressure to start new behaviors that I wasn't committed to or even ready for. Of course, I started to resist, and then withdrew altogether from this change.

Considering what stage you're in may be a game changer for you to successfully modify your behaviors. Breaking down the steps to change your behavior will help you become more focused, specific, and effective. Checking in with yourself and tracking your progress every week will allow you to understand where you've been, where you want to go, and make tiny adjustments to help ensure your success.

PRECONTEMPLATION—I WON'T.

When someone is not even considering adopting a positive or healthy behavior, it's usually because they don't believe they have a problem. If you find yourself in this stage, your family and friends are probably the ones pressuring you to make changes that you just don't agree with. Most likely, you just want the acknowledgment and appreciation that you have full control of your choices. No one particularly likes being judged or made to feel inadequate. Your loved ones are likely irritating you at this point because they are pointing something out that you don't see as a problem.

PRECONTEMPLATION—I CAN'T.

You know you need to address an unhealthy issue, but you're afraid that making this change is too complicated or difficult. You may have even tried and failed once or twice in the past, causing negative emotions to overwhelm you. Maybe you have very low expectations that any changes can really lead to success.

If this sounds familiar, relax. You're in great company. We are all in this stage at some point or other. You deserve genuine empathy and unconditional acceptance, starting with you. Instead of pushing yourself to make a behavior change before you're ready, focus on understanding *why* you want to make this change. I often encourage my clients to use a process called decisional balance—an effective method to weigh the pros and cons of making a behavioral change.

DECISIONAL BALANCE

PROS	CONS
• Why do you want to change this behavior? • What will you gain from making changes?	• Why should you have to change this behavior? • How is your life better if you continue with what you're doing?

1. Do the pros outweigh the cons?
2. What are the obstacles to make this change?
3. What would it take for you to change the behavior and overcome the cons?
4. Can you really do it? (YES!)

I had a client who was having trouble sleeping. She did a little research and came across several articles suggesting that using electronics at bedtime was the likely culprit interfering with her sleep cycles. However, like many of us, she was very attached to her phone. Here's a series of questions and answers we went over together.

How is your life better if you continue with what you're doing? Being on my phone makes me happy. I get to catch up and see what my friends are doing and play games. And there's no absolute proof that the phone affects my sleep. Maybe there are other reasons why I can't sleep.

Why would you want to stop using your phone before bedtime? I haven't actually proved that the blue light doesn't interfere with my sleep, but I haven't been sleeping well this whole year and I'm tired of being tired. Something needs to change.

What is more important? Getting sleep or making yourself happy? Getting sleep would make me very happy!

What are your obstacles to making this change? I LOVE my phone and I've been looking at my phone before bedtime for years! It'll be hard to break this habit.

What alternatives could you try besides looking at your phone right before bedtime? I could look at my phone after dinner instead. I could start a different habit before bedtime that's more soothing, like taking a bath or listening to some music. I could also put my phone in another room to charge so I won't be tempted to look at it.

Can you really do this? It will be hard because I've been doing this for a long time, but I have three different strategies that I can try.

My client discovered other habits that replaced her phone time right before bed. Her sleep quality increased and soon she was able to break her nightly phone time. She definitely had some setbacks—wine was not a good substitute for her, but through trial and error, a positive attitude, and persistence, she was able to keep working on this over six weeks. In the end, not only was she well rested, but she also felt that she had enough confidence to overcome some other bad habits she'd been wanting to break.

By taking the time to really understand the benefits of a new nighttime routine and understanding how the behavior change would benefit her life, she moved herself from the pre-contemplative stage to successfully establishing a relaxing nighttime routine.

CONTEMPLATION—I MAY.

A good portion of this road trip to wellness will be working in the contemplation stage. Just like an actual road trip, the journey may be even more important than the destination. You'll need to discover your strengths and understand your core values to keep yourself motivated and find long-term success.

In this stage, you're beginning to plan how to make the changes you want to see. You're more aware of the benefits and less satisfied with your present health and well-being. You may still have a sense of doubt and find reasons for delaying the change. Part of your feelings may stem from fear, afraid that making the change will be difficult or even impossible to achieve. You're not alone.

People typically remain in the contemplation stage for longer than necessary, weighing the benefits of change against the effort it'll take. It's easy to get hung up on the what-ifs and delay the hard work, but you've got to push past this stage to make any progress to your health and well-being. Consider the pros to making this behavioral change. Connect to your strengths and get excited about the possibilities that could emerge. Relive your past accomplishments and remember what strengths and mindset you used to successfully complete your goals. Pinpointing how you were able to overcome obstacles in the past will help you overcome barriers for this upcoming change.

It's also important to identify the downsides of giving up the old behaviors. Doing so may help you see the pros even better. What is negotiable? What isn't? If you're trying to train for a marathon and you have an active family, you'll have time and energy conflicts. Brainstorm compromises and understand the real value of what this new change might entail.

You might have to modify your plans to work with the important aspects of your life such as spending time with your family, but you won't have to completely give up on anything. Making goals to move past this stage would include doing the research—reading, talking, listening, discovering, and deciding. You could also try little experiments that are along the lines of the change you want to make. This will help build your faith and improve your confidence to make the larger behavioral change.

PREPARATION – I WILL.

It's time to connect the dots between the changes you want to make and what they hold for your future. This information will give you clarity as you start exploring different ideas and taking little actions to try them out. By doing this, you'll be able to discover strong motivators that will keep you moving forward to the next stage.

By now, you have mostly overcome your ambivalence and strengthened your motivation. Now is the time to start planning the action you want to take. You probably have one or more strong motivators, and you know what barriers you might have to overcome. But you also know the possible solutions that can lead you through them to success. Experiment with possible solutions and tweak your plan as necessary—be flexible! You can try several options and create new approaches. Break each change and action into smaller steps with specific details of what, when, and how.

Don't be surprised or disheartened if you're still experiencing a bit of ambivalence, resistance, or fear for this challenge. This is completely normal. When you're feeling this way, explore the reasons behind the feelings and identify new ways to help you navigate around these challenges.

It's also advisable to work out several contingency plans in case the unexpected comes up (Murphy's Law!). If you have a workaround planned out before these obstacles arise, it won't be as stressful or difficult to overcome them. Before any barriers arise, you will already have plans A, B, and C in place. Working them out ahead of time will prevent you from losing that valuable momentum.

TAKE ACTION—I AM.

This stage is all about the action—you are officially embarking on your road trip! As with all travel, you can count on part of it not going as planned. But because you prepared for this before you left home, it's perfectly okay. You're flexible and have created backup plans. Nothing can stop you! As a side bonus, you will build your resiliency as you face these challenges, learn to expect the unexpected, adapt, and persevere despite the hiccups.

During this part of your road trip, you'll be focusing on practicing your new behaviors and maintaining consistency. Start small, like working out just one or two times a week. Continually increase the behavior over time until you reach your target level. This is very important to prevent burnout. Keep your strengths and your core values in mind as you travel within this stage. Make new connections and develop relationships with people who share your interests and behavioral goals.

I'd like to highlight one common challenge that you may face. As you change, your relationships may also. You may find that some of your existing relationships will go through turbulent times. Friends and family may feel threatened and/or left out with your new life, and this may be difficult emotionally. Hang in there despite this bumpy road. Evaluate those relationships and determine if they are really benefiting you. If they aren't, it may be time to cut out the toxins. If they are, make a conscious effort to keep the connection strong, but remain strong for yourself also. You have every right to care for yourself, and someone who truly loves you should be able to respect that.

Keep in mind that all your trips are important learning opportunities, not failures. If one of your day trips included a regular salsa dance class and other commitments often kept you from going, realize that is not a failure. Rather, it's valuable information that lets you know to find something that works better with your schedule, or you may need to make more space for it if this particular thing matters to you.

I also recommended that you provide yourself with some rest stops on your journey. Even when you're on the best road trip, you can still get tired and just want to coast. You're learning new things about yourself, meeting new people, and processing different ideas—it's all good, but it is a lot to take in. An all-or-nothing mentality will lead to guilt, self-blame, and—most devastating—a reason to quit. Set yourself up for success. If you need a break, take it. But don't linger there too long or you may lose momentum. If you find yourself having difficulty leaving the rest stop, consider the reasons behind it and adapt as necessary.

Develop your discussions with yourself to process the setbacks you face and reframe them as sources of valuable lessons. Explore your response to an unexpected hiccup—could you have made a better decision, or what would you do differently next time? Reframing the obstacles as lessons and day trips as experiments will remove that feeling of failure and help you approach life with an openness and curiosity.

MAINTENANCE – I STILL AM.

Imagine coming home from a trip where you did yoga every morning and discovered that you also really like mango. In fact, you liked it so much, you decided to start incorporating it into your normal daily routine. That's what this part of the action stage is like—incorporating the actions you tried and enjoyed into your life to the point that they stop being a goal and become more like a habit. This usually happens six months after you've initiated them. Your confidence is high at this point.

And then the dreaded day comes that throws you off your routine. You get another project tossed in your lap and now you don't have the time to attend your morning yoga class. In addition, there's a mango shortage and you find yourself reaching for that cinnamon roll again. Now you're getting worried. You can see yourself easily abandoning theses healthy behaviors, and after you've worked so hard over the last several months and been successful, this can be very frustrating.

Sometimes in life we have to zag when we're used to zigging. Relapses are challenging and it's important to keep remembering your strengths, values, resources, and vision. Even though it may feel like it, you don't have to start all over again. You've already experienced the value and benefit of yoga and mangos! You're simply in the maintenance stage, which means you can get yourself back on track quickly with little effort. You've got this!

Making lifestyle changes can be challenging, but you can achieve them! You may even find it to be easy once you understand what stage of behavioral change you are in. For me, giving up sugar felt overwhelming, and I admit that I still occasionally go into a chocolate frenzy (usually around the holidays), which means I'm often in maintenance mode. However, knowing this helps me formulate a strategy and make contingency plans to overcome the temptations. While I'm not completely sugar-free, my sugar consumption has gone down considerably and I'm comfortable with that. In fact, my A1C went from 5.9 and to 5.2. I can literally see the results of my hard work, and that keeps me going.

Your road trip is not necessarily going to always be in the action phase. Sometimes, you may jump back into maintenance mode, and that's okay. Similarly, some road trips may take longer than others to reach your destination. If you begin in the precontemplation stage and this journey gets you to the contemplation stage, then I'd consider your road trip a success!

Often times, we crave visible proof like losing ten pounds or running a half-marathon. Those things are all very rewarding, but so is making a decision to do that thing you've always wanted to do and sticking to it despite the pesky obstacles that keep getting in the way. By understanding the specific behavioral stages, you can realize what an accomplishment it is to move yourself beyond one stage and into the next one, especially if you've been there for a long time.

I always knew I had an issue with sugar, but it probably took me over five years to do something about it—it just felt so daunting, and I didn't know where to start. Once I did some soul searching and understood what stage I was in, the specific goal was to get myself beyond it and progress forward. I wasn't focused on giving up sugar, and I was done berating myself endlessly for my lack of willpower and discipline. But to succeed, I had to understand and connect to the reasons I wanted to give up sugar. I needed to start small and design strategies to help conquer this addiction and remain focused on the end goal. I did the cha-cha, going weeks without sugar and then binging on chocolate. Finally, it became a habit to pass on dessert rather than a forced refrain. But at times when I do indulge, I have to put in the effort to not continue the backward spiral. Keeping my vision and whys front and center helps to make this journey easier.

There is light at the end of the tunnel for you too. With self-compassion, a plan, and a vision, you will be able to travel to a healthier you!

WHAT TO PACK

"Our battered suitcases were piled on the
sidewalk again; we had longer ways to go.
But no matter, the road is life."
– Jack Kerouac

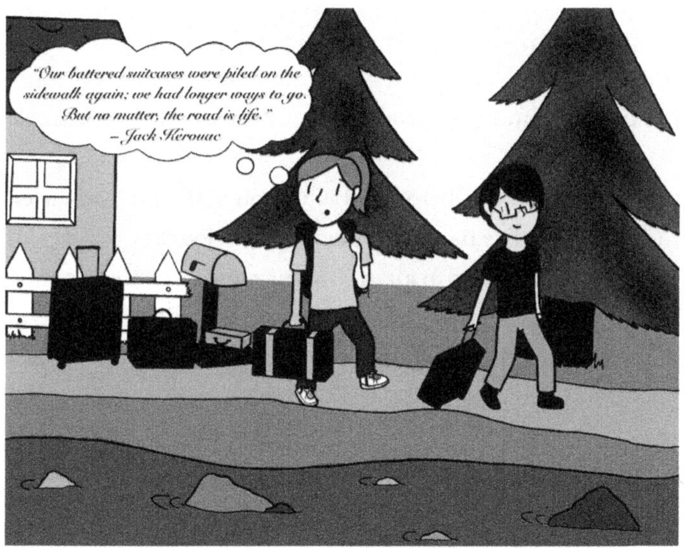

I don't know about you, but it's taken me forty-five years to finally learn how to pack properly. I would mentally plan what I needed to bring as I was booking the trip. Then I would obsessively look at blogs and shop online for the perfect travel outfits, shoes, and accessories. Finally, the night before, I would take my suitcase out and start stuffing all those things in my carry-on bag. I'd quickly realize I wouldn't be able to take everything I planned to, so I would start to negotiate with my inner fashionista and wannabe beauty influencer and pack just the survivors. Even after sacrificing a lot of items, I'd often find during the trip that I only needed half of what I brought!

It's normal to think that you need everything packed and ready before you take yourself through this road trip to wellness. You will want to clear your calendar, sign up for those fitness classes, finish all your work projects, wait until after Aunt Jennie comes in July, and it might help if you lost those pesky ten pounds before you start walking in the mornings.

Of course, if you're being real with yourself, you don't need to do any of that before you begin your journey. In fact, if you wait for the stars to align, you may never step one foot on your road trip. Start NOW—there's no time like the present! Cultivate the four most essential items and get moving!

ESSENTIAL ITEMS FOR SUCCESS

CLEAR INTENTION

We talked about setting your vision earlier, but now I'd like you to obtain clarity for your intentions. I recently listened to a wonderful podcast with Brendon Burchard, a successful performance coach, and he emphasized asking better questions to get better answers. When you're 100% clear on why you want to do something, you become more proactive, gain momentum, and understand your reasons every step of the way.

It also helps to be clear about who you would like to be during this journey. Define how you'd like to show up and what words will remind you of the person you want to be. Stop for a moment and come up with three words that define your best self. These could be your VIA character strengths (remember the survey we discussed earlier?) or words that connect to your values and your vision. Consider words like compassion, loyalty, forgiveness, honesty, perseverance, and leadership. Feel free to Google "character strengths" to come up with some more ideas.

Keeping your three words in mind, make it a daily habit to ask yourself the following clarity questions. It's okay if you find that your answers change a bit as you get farther along in the process. This means you're growing and evolving, and that's good! By revisiting these questions on a regular basis, you'll be able to clarify your vision and reflect on what you're feeling from day to day.

CLEAR INTENTION

1. What three words would you use to describe your best self?

2. Why do you want to make this change?

3. Why has this been so difficult to change in the past? What pain/fear do you associate with this change?

4. What will it cost you if you don't make this change?

5. Are you willing to do what it takes to have this change be successful?

One of my clients wanted to increase her well-being. For the last thirty years, she was a department head at her job and found that she had lost sight of what really mattered to her— her family, herself, and her happiness. While she didn't want to quit her job, she did want to start making major changes in her life to support her new vision. However, her reputation of "always getting things done" allowed constant interruptions and emergencies to block her path, making it difficult for her to reconnect with her family and get that much-needed "me" time. This was challenging. Not only did she need to change her usual approach, but she also needed to help the people she worked with understand that she was no longer accessible 24/7.

What really helped this client was the daily routine of going through the clear intention questionnaire above. The three words she chose for her best self were compassion, love, and boundaries. These words made her priorities and intentions clear and sealed her commitment to become that version of herself. That's not to say that she started turning everyone away to maintain her boundaries. Sometimes she had be flexible and make exceptions. However, instead of automatically canceling her personal time and family events like in the past, she was able to better determine how to prioritize what really mattered over things that could wait. This demonstrated to her loved ones that she was serious about spending quality time with them.

Clarifying your intentions on a daily basis will help you discover what skills you need to make your change. For this client, she was able to refine her negotiating skills, strengthen her personal boundaries, and work on tactful communication. She learned how to say no with compassion and choose the person she wanted to become. It's not enough to have intention. You need to commit to your intentions and be clear that the qualities of your best self and purpose in life are tied to your well-being.

MINDFULNESS

Another essential item to pack is mindfulness. Becoming more mindful through meditation was a game changer for me. I can honestly tell you that it guided me to a happier and healthier place. Before I started meditating, I was one of those people who would scream at other drivers, scowl when I wasn't happy with a situation, and often walked around in such a funk that my family was afraid to even come near me.

Today's way of life puts you in a constant stress mode. There are deadlines and appointments galore, booking your calendar out for two weeks at a time and making you feel stretched to the limit. Sometimes it feels like everybody and everything needs something from you. As I like to say, "I just need to slow the treadmill down." You have control over your life—you can slow down the treadmill of life and control the pace.

Doing so is scary and will be a challenge. You will have to face all the thoughts you're running from. When you are constantly busy, you go on autopilot. This makes it easier to avoid worries, concerns, and issues. But even if you don't make the deliberate choice to face your fears, they always find a way to catch up with you, don't they? So, why not maintain the control and slow down your treadmill?

MEDITATION

Mindfulness often comes hand-in-hand with meditation, an excellent way to slow down your treadmill. According to an article on the Positive Psychology website, some of the "oldest documented images of meditation are from India and date back to 5,000 [or] 3,500 BCE" (Mead, "Meditation."). Meditation has a long tradition in Hinduism, although you can also see influence from many other religions such as Buddhism, Judaism, and Islam. Some even view the Christian prayer as a form of meditation.

Usually people are seated during meditation, but you can also meditate while walking or lying on your bed. The beauty of meditation is you can customize it to your ever-changing needs. The main point is to take yourself away from the chaotic parts of your life and just be quiet. It's an intentional practice in which you focus to increase calmness, concentration, awareness, and emotional balance. During this quiet time, you'll perform some deep breathing and maintain awareness of your breath, consciously guiding your mind toward an anchor or a single point of focus. This time is used to turn inward. Whether you do it for five minutes or an hour, you'll give yourself a much-needed reset and should then be able to calmly go about your day.

Although meditation and mindfulness are often performed together, they have very different purposes. While meditation is the actual activity of finding stillness in the midst of chaos, mindfulness is about living in the present moment. Mindfulness gives you the chance to notice what's going on around you and acknowledge your thoughts, feelings, behaviors, movements, and the impact you have on others.

You can practice mindfulness by being fully engaged in the present moment. Unlike meditation where it's best to find a quiet area, you can apply mindfulness with everything you do. Making coffee, walking your dog, watching a movie, talking with your best friend—it's all about focusing what is happening in that very moment. You can do this anywhere, with anyone, and at any time.

Being present takes WORK! Recently, I caught myself not being mindful during a conversation with my partner. While he was talking, my mind was clearly not on the conversation, and understandably, this was frustrating for him. It is so easy to have a sense of disconnect in the world we live in, especially with all of the electronics constantly dinging with alerts and pulling our attention away from the moment.

But learning to take notice of the present moment will help you understand the value of the process. Mindfulness can help you feel more connected and enjoy quality relationships, along with giving you clarity, focus, improved memory, and more. For example, if you were only fixated on the number on your scale while trying to lose weight, you wouldn't notice the wonderful healthy habits that you adopt in the process. You wouldn't notice how much more you incorporate exercise into your daily routine. You wouldn't notice how you set the bag of chips down when you practiced your breathing exercises. You wouldn't notice the increased quality of life that you're living.

Being aware of the present allows you to realize that the outcome isn't the only important factor on your road trip to wellness. You can enjoy and appreciate all the moments that take place *during* your travels also. Ralph Waldo Emerson is attributed with saying, "Life is a journey, not a destination." You need to remember to appreciate the process as well as the results.

When I started practicing mindfulness, I noticed that I was losing my critical judgment of both myself and others. I can't tell you how often those negative thoughts would derail my goals. When I was giving up sugar and would succumb to a cookie or sweet, I'd beat myself up and just quit my quest. When I learned to let go of the judgment and instead allow compassion for myself during my struggles, I was able to shake off the minor setback and do better the next day.

I believe you will find meditation and mindfulness incredibly useful on your road trip. You might be facing some pretty deep challenges, and these tools will prove beneficial. I recommend you perform daily time-outs to clear your mind before facing a challenge. As you're adopting new habits and getting rid of old ones, mindfulness will be key to awakening your understanding of the process and ultimately finding success.

Let's say that one of your destinations/goals is to eat a healthier diet. You're used to working through lunch and usually your body is nagging at you to feed it. So, you end up grabbing anything you see and stuff it down in under a minute before continuing with your day. You did the best you could on autopilot, but let's see what happens when you apply principles from meditation and mindfulness.

You have a hectic day, but you also have a fifteen-minute break. You take five of those minutes to shut your office door and do some deep breathing, only focusing on your breath. After you're done, you find yourself feeling much more relaxed and ready to work toward your goal to eat healthier. On your lunch break, you are happy that you brought a healthy lunch. You enjoy every bite of your food, taking in the whole experience—the sounds, the tastes, the textures. At the end of your short lunch, you feel refreshed and ready to face the next phone call, conference, or meeting.

See the difference that meditation and mindfulness can make? The beauty is that they don't have to take a huge chunk out of your day. If you're consistent with daily sessions, even if they're short, you'll see the difference. You'll find that the benefits will last the whole day, week, month, and even year. You're giving your mind a well-deserved rest and training it to focus on the important things and letting others go.

As you become more familiar with meditation and mindfulness, you might consider taking it further and practicing the combined ritual of mindfulness meditation. This method teaches how to be unconditionally present, no matter what is happening. I reached a new level with these principles—they help me accept the reality of what life is in each present moment. It helps me learn how to trust my own inherent wisdom and not spin my wheels by wishing things were different. It aids me in facing discomfort, experiencing constant changes, and building faith that things will work out the way they are supposed to. Knowing that you will have highs and lows, mindfulness meditation can teach you to be content and grateful to experience life just the way it is.

I highly recommend that you incorporate mindfulness meditation into your life. The benefits will far outweigh the ten minutes it'll take you each day. It'll leave you feeling refreshed and ready to take on whatever life throws at you with contentment and resilience. Learning to be present without judgment will bring you a sense of peace.

A YOGI'S APPROACH

So many people are afraid of yoga because they can't touch their toes or do the elaborate poses they see on Instagram. I can tell you as a fifty-nine-year-old woman, headstands and extreme backbends are out of my practice. They just don't feel good anymore, and that's the beauty of yoga—you are encouraged to modify to your comfort level and abilities. If you find difficulty balancing, you can just put your foot on the ground or grab a wall. You can use a strap if you can't reach your foot, and you can use blankets or blocks to make the poses more comfortable.

This is the biggest takeaway from yoga—you are encouraged to adjust a pose or action to accommodate your body, mind, and spirit to where you are in the present moment. You get to choose. If your goal is to do a yoga class but you're completely exhausted, you can choose to lie in a restorative pose and still be achieving your goal.

Believe it or not, you don't have to get on the mat to have a yogi's approach to life. No pretzel bending or headstands required! You can apply the modification concept to your whole life. For example, if you've had a rough day, you may not feel up to being super active with your kids, but you could sit on the couch and read them a story. It's okay to have an off day and take the simpler route from time to time. The thing to remember is to strive to keep these as exceptions and not the norm. Always give your best effort to achieve your original goal, but understand that when life happens, you do have the choice to modify or find alternatives and still accomplish your objectives.

When I signed up for my yoga teacher's certification, I had fears that I would be expected to bend in ways my body did not want to. I quickly learned that what I thought of as yoga was only a small part of this wonderful way of living. There are many more aspects to yoga that have nothing to do with the physical poses (known as asanas). It's more about a way of living and approaching life, integrating your mind, body, and spirit to bring contentment and peace.

For one of my class assignments, I read *The Heart of Yoga* by T.K.V. Desikachar. In his book, he mentions how yoga was established in 3,000 BC and derived from the six fundamental Indian systems known collectively as darsana. Darsana is a specific way of seeing, almost like looking inside yourself as though through a mirror. It creates opportunities for you to better recognize yourself.

According to Desikachar, the definition of yoga is "to tie the strands of the mind together." What this means is that yoga starts in your mind before doing the physical work. Another meaning he provides is "to attain what was previously unattainable." If we want to do something differently, we must go through the process of learning, changing, and growing to become who we want to be. Every change is considered yoga, and we can gain more understanding of ourselves and others, reaching a point we've never been before.

Yoga is also about focusing all your attention on the activity that you're currently engaging in. The more focused you are, the greater attentiveness to your actions in each present moment. The advantage of this focus is you get better and better each time. An amazing aspect of yoga is you can begin from any starting point by consciously incorporating all aspects of yourself (mind, body, and spirit), and you do this step by step. You are not tied to your bad habits—every day and every action will be fresh rather than thoughtless repetition.

Centuries ago, there was a wise Indian sage named Patanjali who laid out a guide (just like this one!) to help his followers chart their course to contentment. It contained essential advice for daily living. Patanjali's guide, known as the Yoga Sutras, was specifically designed to lead to greater happiness and fulfillment.

AVIDYA

An important concept from Patanjali is avidya, meaning incorrect comprehension or false perception. Avidya teaches how perception and action can get you into trouble. You may be unconsciously dependent on habits that don't serve you and could even be harmful. I used to love having coffee with my mother. She always enjoyed a cookie or sweet to accompany her coffee, and I learned to do the same. Unfortunately, as someone who is at a high risk for diabetes, this habit was harmful to my well-being.

Likewise, you need to understand that your perceptions are not necessarily true or real. Sometimes it's easy to assess a situation based on your history and beliefs rather than being open to new possibilities. Using the yogi's approach, avidya obscures your clarity of consciousness with a filmy layer, and sometimes this can be hard to recognize. However, there are some characteristics or branches that you *can* recognize and use your awareness of them to your advantage.

AVIDYA BRANCHES

Ego – This pushes you into thinking you need to be better than other people. "I know that I'm right."

Making Demands/Desires – The desire for things that you don't really need. It's never enough.

Pure Rejection – Letting your past experiences cause you to assume similar situations will bring you pain again. You reject anything that is a difficult experience.

Fear – Having doubts and fighting against uncertainty. You prefer to continue with the familiar path, blocking out new opportunities.

Being consciously aware that these obstacles will cloud your perceptions and make you dissatisfied can help you tap into who you are and what you truly need or want. Can you imagine taking this road trip and feeling zero tension, unrest, or agitation? Tapping inside yourself and sensing where the quietness is within you can help bring you clarity and peace.

PARINAMAVADA

It's also important to understand that everything is in a constant state of flux. This concept of continual change is known as parinamavada. The way you see things today does not have to be the same as you saw it yesterday, or even the same way you will see it tomorrow.

I have a client who, after spending most of her adult life in various relationships, was just going through her fourth divorce during one of our meetings. She was discouraged and determined that she was going to live her life on her own from here on out, but this was a foreign concept for her and would take adjustment. She decided to go to therapy. I watched the healing transformation as she started making time for herself and her own interests.

She later told me that she met someone in her hiking group and her interest was piqued. "He's completely charming and I love hiking with him. But I think he's getting too interested, so I need to back off. I'm not good with relationships—my divorces are proof."

We transitioned from there to another subject, but the conversation came back around to her new hiking friend. It was clear she wanted the relationship to be a little more than just a hiking buddy, and so I asked her, "Do you think you're the same person you were last year?"

She immediately answered, "Oh god, no. I'm so much more grounded and such a better communicator. Plus, I've really made my work schedule more reasonable, and now I have time to do the things I enjoy. My mood is better, and I feel great." There was a long quiet moment as she soaked in what I was trying to get across.

My client ended up asking her hiking buddy to lunch after one of their hikes and, while she's not eagerly running to the altar, she is enjoying her first real relationship in which she knows herself. She realized that she is a different person today than in her past relationships. Everything, including herself, is constantly changing, which means any future relationships and possibilities are changing also.

Practicing self-reflection and disseminating what is accurate versus a spiral of false thoughts is part of the yogi's practice. You can never be sure of the outcome of your actions. By letting go of your expectations and paying attention to the actions themselves, you can achieve yoga as a state of being. You can change your approach, actions, and outcomes.

The purpose of yoga is to unify your actions—to be aware of what is happening in the present, to focus more on the process than the result, to filter through your false perceptions, to work through your avidya branches, and to understand that change is constant. These are all wonderful pieces of knowledge that you can bring along when you're on your road trip to wellness. This is a great opportunity to incorporate self-reflection and truthfulness in your perspective. Keep checking in with yourself to be sure that your beliefs are accurate and realistic. Our minds can be deceiving. As mentioned earlier, this is often called monkey mind in meditation, but you can work on training yourself to recognize and move past this.

Let me allow you to witness an example of monkey mind in my own personal history. One day while cleaning out my closet, I quickly found how easy it is to become distracted. It started off innocent enough but come with me and watch as I spiral into darkness and self-judgment.

"Oh, I remember when I bought this dress! I was so excited to wear it."

"Now, it just looks like I'm trying to be a teenager. It's really snug."

"I'm just not the same as I used to be. Why can't things just stay the same?"

"It's because I have no self-discipline. I knew I shouldn't have had dessert last night."

"I'm ashamed of myself. I can't do anything right."

"I might as well stick to home and never go out. It's much safer just watching TV and hanging with my dogs."

See how quickly that spiraled? The sad thing is, while there was a bit of *reality* in my thoughts, there wasn't a lot of *truth*. The reality was I had been excited to wear the dress ten years ago, but things had changed since then. The truth was that dress was no longer my style—it was snug because my shoulders had gotten bigger from practicing yoga (I was making my body stronger!). I did have dessert the night prior (reality), but I've cut my sugar intake drastically, and I only took one bite off someone else's plate (truth). Did I really feel like I couldn't do anything right? Of course not, I was just disappointed that one of my favorite dresses wasn't right for me anymore. It's okay to mourn changes, but you also need to recognize the truths behind those changes.

AHIMSA

There's another principle in yoga called ahimsa, which means acting toward all living beings with love, genuine care, and compassion, while refraining from harming any creatures in your mind, speech, or actions. This care extends to yourself.

As you journey on this road trip, it is essential to practice ahimsa toward yourself. You will be in a new environment, and you may be a little wobbly and unsure of yourself. You'll have to brave new approaches and accept uncovered truths that might make you uncomfortable. Taking a vow of ahimsa and pledging to practice love and compassion toward yourself and to those around you will make this road trip far easier and more enjoyable.

Yogis will always adjust their poses to fit within what they can handle at that time—there is no self-judgment about it. Applying this approach to your road trip will reinforce the mindset that you are going on a journey—it's a process, an adventure, a learning curve. Things that you thought would work may not. Unexpected hiccups will appear. This is all perfectly normal, and you should expect and welcome these unplanned occurrences as nothing more than learning experiences and information.

How many times have our happy accidents or plan Bs turned out to be the best experiences or the most memorable part of our trip? That is truly the meaning of the yogi's approach—experiencing the whole process of the journey. Your endgame isn't to simply perfect a headstand or make it through that 108-degree hot yoga class. It's about discovering the person you become on the journey. When you allow yourself to think about who and where you are in life, you will accept the present realities and still point your compass toward the ideal.

RESILIENCE

When it comes to travel, I've missed several planes, been surprised by the rainstorm that wasn't predicted in the weather report and had to scroll frantically through my Expedia app when I forgot to make a hotel reservation for the day we landed. Your ability to recover from the hiccups affects your physical and mental health and the quality of your relationships. It truly is the basic ingredient to happiness and success. However, it's common to not be emotionally or psychologically prepared for adversity. This makes it easy for you to give up on the things you truly want.

It's effortless to stick to your routine—it's familiar and comfortable, you know what to expect, and there's no stress over changes. In general, there's nothing wrong with a regular routine. But what if it narrows your perspective and prevents you from doing something that you really want to do? That's when you need to call upon your resilience.

Resilience seems to be the new buzzword lately and I think it really deserves the hype it's getting. The ability to adapt when plans don't go the way you hoped or expected demonstrates that resilience is the key to success in anything you do. It goes hand-in-hand with perseverance and success. The beauty of life is that you can boost your resilience with some slight shifts on how you think about adversity. You can even beef up the strength of your resilience and learn skills that will help you understand the "how and why" to the way you think. Resilience is a mindset that will enable you to seek out new experiences and view your life as a work-in-progress.

At some point in our lives, most of us have come up against a major obstacle, some life-altering event that may have blown you way off course. Maybe it was the death of a loved one, the loss of a job, the breakup of a long-term relationship, or another event that brought you trauma and setback. The negative memories tax your resilience and often cause you to become fearful and feel helpless. But you can learn to bounce back and find a way to move forward. You can strengthen your resilience.

Have you ever looked up to someone who appears to have it all? From the outside, it can seem like their life just fell into their laps. They have a great career, perfect relationships, and enviable skills and passions—they are so lucky! But likely, they worked hard for the life they have, and continually work hard to maintain it. Research has shown that these things require a combination of desire and character. If you want it strongly enough, you can develop your resilience and obtain it. Openness and a commitment to live an enriched and meaningful life is key on this adventure.

The psychology field has worked tirelessly to determine what factors enable people to bounce back and thrive despite their obstacles. They discovered three main traits that contribute to resilience.

ASSESSING RISK

Your confidence in your own ability to assess risk and deal with the obstacles that stand in your way will provide you with a safety net when you reach for your goals. When you have faith in your ability to respond to uncertainty, pursuing your goals becomes less scary. If you are realistically optimistic and forecasting with accuracy, your plan Bs (or alternative strategies) will help you handle any obstacles or potential problems that may come up. You can have faith things will work out in the end, even if they don't go exactly as planned. But you need to buy in to the understanding that there is never just ONE path to get to your destination.

EMOTIONAL INTELLIGENCE

People who have a keen sense of themselves and are comfortable expressing their thoughts and feelings can use their emotional awareness to track subtle signs in the receptiveness of others. This strong interpersonal skill enables lasting relationships with yourself and others, helping you know when to push forward and when to stop. Knowing yourself allows you to determine if there's a true fit between the people you're trying to work with and what they may be experiencing.

Not all pursuits are realistic, and an emotionally intelligent person can understand this. They know when to pull back and when to persevere, and they don't feel any shame or sense of failure when it's the former. Being confident in your ability to assess risk and problem solve when you hit obstacles provides you with a safety net that makes it easier to pursue new experiences and forge new relationships. When you have faith in your ability to respond to the uncertain, moving forward toward your goal becomes less daunting.

PURPOSE

Show me a resilient person and I'll bet their pursuits are motivated by a strong and meaningful purpose. Purpose requires a focus on the present. No matter how long it takes, a person with a strong sense of purpose will stick to their mission. They've found value in what they're doing and that helps them see the complete picture.

Reaching out of your comfort zone is risky. It takes a good amount of courage and inner strength. You risk rejection and failure, and that's scary! But there's a big payoff if you can remain strong. Building your resilience has many benefits in addition to helping you reach your goals. By becoming more resilient, you'll improve your ability to assess risk and plan for potential problems. You'll deepen your emotional awareness and your connections. You'll become more mindful and start to discover the meaning in your life. The best part is you can start building your resiliency RIGHT NOW!

Let's discuss seven aspects to start incorporating into your daily life to build up your resiliency.

MINDFUL RESPONSES TO ADVERSE SITUATIONS

Your emotions and behaviors are triggered not by events themselves, but by how you're interpreting those events. These interpretations stem from how you feel about yourself and your past experiences. Start listening to your inner thoughts when faced with an adverse situation. Identify how your thoughts can affect your feelings and behavior.

Biology plays another big part in how we react. Our brains are hardwired to survive. The amygdala is part of the limbic system, and its primary role is generating and storing emotions. The hippocampus stores these facts, and our neocortex helps us process the emotions and facts. Many times, when our emotions get the better of us, the amygdala overrides this process and mobilizes our fear to get us out of danger. Do you ever find yourself overreacting to something that you feel should be considered insignificant in your overall perspective? When emotions cloud our thinking, it's difficult to shift out of our emotional mode and into our rational thinking mode.

You must understand the emotional impact of how these reactions can be counterproductive and cloud your thinking. In doing so, you'll be able to understand what you are feeling and why you're feeling that way. Using this knowledge, you'll be able to put the brakes on your emotions, calm yourself, and focus on how to solve the issue that's blocking your way or come up with an alternative.

AVOID THINKING TRAPS

Your five senses can take in much more information than your brain can process at one time. Sometimes the information gets simplified and doesn't get properly processed. The brain cuts corners and takes shortcuts to keep up with the sensory overload, which means you're not getting a realistic or direct readout of what is actually happening. And, of course, with your amygdala stepping in at every opportunity to protect you, it's easy to miss important information and get trapped in your thinking. Don't feel bad, this is very human. In fact, there are eight common thinking traps that will interfere with our resilience and how we handle the setbacks and stresses in our daily lives.

THINKING TRAPS

Jumping to Conclusions – Making assumptions without the relevant data. Understand that there may be certain situations that automatically make you vulnerable to this trap. Force yourself to pause before you fall for it.

Tunnel Vision – Selectively focusing on positive or negative outcomes. This is connected with your strong belief about yourself and your world. You only screen information that's consistent with your beliefs and ignore the data that could disconfirm them.

Magnifying and Minimizing – Focusing too much on either the positives or the negatives of a situation. Magnifying the negatives and minimizing the positives can lead to a negative mood and compromised resilience. But the opposite—magnifying the positive and minimizing the negative—may cause you to underestimate the real need for a life change. Resilience rests on an accurate appraisal of your life.

Personalizing – Blaming yourself. This thinking trap is the reflex tendency to attribute problems to your own doing. Interestingly enough, many psychologists will point out that if you attribute the cause of the problem to yourself, you also grant yourself the power to solve it. Whether you perceive the control of your life as coming from within or from an outside force—such as others, luck, or circumstances—determines how resilient you are. Resiliency results from the belief that *you* have the power to control the events in your life and can change what needs changing.

Externalizing – Blaming others. This thinking trap is the opposite of personalizing. If you think problems or situations are rarely your fault, you're simply blaming outside forces whenever something goes wrong. Not realizing that an adversity is genuinely of your own doing or within your control may cause you to find yourself prone to anger and disappointment as you feel out of control of the situation at hand.

Overgeneralizing – Not taking into account all the factors involved. When personalizers overgeneralize, they assassinate their own characters. When externalizers overgeneralize, they assassinate the character of others. Both are attributing the causes of problems to character rather than the actual behavior. Neither of these perceptions are motivating. Next time a situation happens, ask yourself, "What behavior—mine or someone else's—could have caused this problem?" Being realistic and open to the truth is the key to resolving the issue and moving forward.

Mind Reading – Assuming we can all read each other's minds. Often, we believe we know what those around us are thinking. Likewise, you might expect others to know what you're thinking. In both scenarios, you fall into the first thinking trap—jumping to conclusions that are rarely full of truth! If you act on this possibly faulty information, it can result in negative feelings and strained relationships.

Emotional Reasoning – Drawing conclusions about the nature of the world based on your emotional state. If a threat seems distant in time, your anxiety is typically low enough to be an insufficient incentive to stop. However, as time goes on and the proximity of the threat becomes closer, your heightened anxiety will falsely inform you that the threat is stronger. This often results in succumbing to emotional reasoning.

So, what are some ways to avoid falling victim to the thinking traps? Check in with reality by using the following thinking trap questions.

THINKING TRAPS

1. Are you certain of these facts or are you just guessing?
2. What's the big picture of the entire situation?
3. Is there a specific behavior that explains this situation?
4. Are you overlooking any positives? Are you overlooking any negatives?
5. What contributed to this situation? What percentage is within your control and what percentage is external?

6. Did you make your feelings and position known clearly? Are you expecting the other person to work hard at figuring out what you want?

7. What questions must you ask the other person to know the facts?

UNDERSTANDING YOUR UNDERLYING BELIEFS

Have you ever overreacted when faced with an adverse situation? Certain intense emotions may arise from time to time, and it can be hard to keep your behavior in check. This is a sign that you're being impacted by an underlying belief. These are deeply held beliefs about how the world ought to be and how you feel you should be within that world.

Underlying beliefs are fixed ideas that often overgeneralize the negative aspects such as people can't be trusted, the world is a dangerous place, being successful is what matters most, you need people to like you, or you always have to be in charge.

Deep motivations and values often drive your actions and goals. These factors determine how you respond to adversity. By becoming aware of and understanding your core values and motivations, you'll be better able to regulate your emotions and improve your empathy toward others. You'll understand what makes you "tick," and better yet, what makes other people "tock."

Your underlying beliefs can minimize your ability to respond to challenging situations, but some others can help you behave in ways that will bring success and happiness. Being honest, showing people respect and dignity, and not giving up when things are difficult will serve you well in multiple facets of your life.

Start identifying your underlying beliefs. "Why" questions have a tendency to put us on the defense, especially when you're required to give a reason why you believe or feel a certain way. It's easy to feel challenged or picked on, and you may end up spending more energy defending your belief rather than working to understand it.

Next time you find yourself in a situation where your underlying beliefs are interfering with reality, strive to stay away from the why and focus more specifically on the what and how. What underlying belief motivates you? What underlying belief makes you afraid? How do they help? What do they cost?

Now that you're aware of some underlying beliefs that might impair your resiliency, the next step is to help yourself break the pattern of reinterpreting or distorting an event to make it fit your underlying belief or applying a confirmation bias. This happens when you start noticing and remembering everything that confirms your belief.

Discovering your underlying beliefs can be a little uncomfortable and unnerving, but I urge you to keep working on it. Once you become aware of what they are, you'll be able to clarify your values and identify what aspects interfere with your ability to respond to adversity effectively. Until then, this core set of beliefs will continue to affect your mood and behavior over and over again. Understanding what is really behind those underlying beliefs will help you figure out when you want to work on changing the beliefs that are getting in your way.

CHALLENGING YOUR BELIEFS

You have the freedom to choose to accept yourself as you are and continue down the same path you've been traveling. However, just the fact that you've made it this far in this book tells me that you are looking to change up your life in exchange for something more fulfilling. This may entail honing skills that can help create that change.

You've learned that viewing the world from a different perspective can open you up to a more accurate view. You've also learned that it is beneficial to be less at the mercy of your emotions and behaviors, and how to work on this so you can respond differently when adverse events occur. Now it's time to ask yourself if you have any lingering beliefs about the futility or difficulty of change.

When you're trying to learn something new or change an old behavior, what is your belief about the possibility of change? If you subscribe to the "you can't teach an old dog new tricks" rule, then I have bad news for you—you're setting yourself up for failure. However, if you were able to uncover your underlying beliefs that play a role in how you feel and behave, the next step is to evaluate how realistic those beliefs are and what you'd like to change so they become more accurate.

The next time adversity strikes, observe your first gut-reaction response. We typically ask ourselves the "why" questions. "Why did this happen?" (Interestingly, we rarely ask why when something good happens). We automatically believe that the cause of the adversity is our responsibility.

If this is true for you, take a deep breath. It's that "pesky" human thing again. In terms of survival, your brain is hard-wired to figure out how to terminate or prevent negative situations, but you can't solve problems without locating the cause. Your brain likes to take shortcuts to process information, which isn't always accurate. And if you identify the wrong cause, you'll pursue the wrong solution.

So, let's change your response. Instead of going directly to why, define the who, what, when, and where (just the facts, ma'am). Avoid the thinking traps we discussed earlier and start focusing more on the what.

CHALLENGING YOUR BELIEFS

1. What underlying belief is kicking in right now? Is it accurate?

2. What is within your control?

3. What is out of your control?

4. What is an ideal solution for this issue?

5. What is a realistic solution for this issue?

6. What can you be flexible about?

7. What beliefs do you need to honor?

PUTTING THINGS IN PERSPECTIVE

Often, I'll wake up in the middle of the night with my mind so revved up, and despite everything I try, I can't get my brain to shut down. Usually, it's because I'm catastrophizing. I'm dwelling on a specific adversity, and within minutes, a chain of disastrous events has replayed over and over in the movie of my mind.

When I became aware of this, the next time it happened, I specifically focused on what was causing me the most worry. Remember, our brains are hardwired (especially at 3 a.m.) to prepare us for a threat that it perceives is heading our way. However, learning to put things in perspective can bring your anxiety down to a manageable level. It can guide you to more accurate thinking.

This approach is designed to change your beliefs about the future. It can help you identify realistic and genuine threats and increase your resilience by regulating your emotions, impulse control, and creating realistic optimism. Try this simple process the next time you see yourself starting to catastrophize.

PROBLEM SOLVING IN ADVERSITY

Problem – When something derails you from your original plan.

You've been very good with your diet lately, except for last night when you gave in to that glass or two of wine.

Three Threats – List your top three threats that could result.

You can't control yourself, you're going to get diabetes, and you're going to die a miserable death.

Probabilities – Estimate the probability of those threats becoming a reality.

Either you'll gain control or keep losing control (50%). If you continue, you'll probably get diabetes, but if you get back on track, you might not (25%). If you do get diabetes and you don't do anything about it, you'll die, but if you do something about it, you'll be able to manage it (10%).

Best Case Alternatives – Generate best case alternatives.

You didn't feel good last night after the wine. Maybe it was good that this happened so you know how poorly you can feel after. You can get to the bottom of why you lose control. Maybe there's something about your underlying beliefs that undermines your willpower. You'll be able to understand what is really happening when you go off your diet and be able to offset the situation the next time something happens.

Problem Solve – And finally, problem solve!

You will investigate what led to you giving into that glass of wine even when you had committed to this diet. You might design a different diet that allows you to go off of it every now and then. You will learn what causes you to go off track and take steps to help you avoid this same situation in the future.

By going through these steps, you'll be able to understand the causes of your setbacks and build your resilience. Instead of an anxiety-filled night, you'll be able to outline strategies that will help you find calmness and refocus your emotions to help support yourself instead of making you fearful. This is a great tool for the heat of the moment, and pretty soon, you'll automatically turn to this approach when adversity strikes.

CALMING EMOTIONS AND CLEARING YOUR THOUGHTS

I'll be honest with you, there is nothing like a stressful situation to make my mind come alive and my body ready for action. In fact, sometimes I'll go in search of situations that would allow me to use my quick action thinking and reflexes. However, doing this too often won't build your resilience, but rather will wear you down and make you ineffective. After a while, your emotions get the better of you and the "itty bitty shitty" voice will start to chatter about all the things that could go wrong.

Chronic stress, runaway emotions, and endless internal chatter drain your resilience reserves. And if you're constantly feeling this, you'll find that your memory and concentration will disappear, as well as create serious issues in your relationships and everyday life. So, how can you find your bearings when your brain hijacks your emotions and increases your stress levels?

Changing the way you think and incorporating calming techniques can help you control how your body and mind respond to stress. You can teach yourself how to get into a state of relaxation. Think about it—the body cannot be stressed and relaxed at the same time. So, if you train yourself to relax, you can control the amount of stress you experience.

CALMING TECHNIQUES

Controlled Breathing – When you're under stress, you start breathing quick, shallow breaths. When you make yourself breathe slowly and deeply, you calm your nervous system down. Focusing on your breaths will give your brain time to determine if this is a real threat or just something that's out of the ordinary.

Progressive Muscle Relaxation – Consciously tensing and relaxing your muscles systematically throughout your body will help change your focus. It will also send signals to your brain that you're not in real danger and there's no need to activate the fight or flight system.

Positive Imagery – There are a lot of jokes about finding your "happy place," but don't discount the effectiveness of creating and relaxing in an image where you are at ease, comfortable, and happy. The more detailed and vivid your visualization is, the more powerful it will be in helping you to relax.

Prepare – Preparing for an upcoming stressor involves positive imagery, but this time in a preventive manner. Let's say you're trying to drink less, but you're currently out on a girls' night. Your friends will notice that you're not drinking as much as you usually do and will comment on it. Will that pressure you into giving up your goal? What happens if you start telling them what you're hoping to gain from drinking less? Most of our friends want to support us, and you might find a more positive outcome than you'd expect by simply being honest.

Mental Games – Challenging yourself to quick mental games (no more than two minutes) can help shift your attention away from those distracting thoughts so you can continue dealing with the task at hand (i.e., the stressful situation). Recite your favorite song lyrics with catchy tunes to put yourself in a good mood. Repeat your favorite uplifting mantra. Select a word and see how many rhymes you can come up with. Anything that will make you refocus will help to rid your mind of any intrusive thoughts.

I recommend that you start practicing these techniques during the quiet times—maybe in the shower or right before going to bed. The more you practice, the better you'll be at shifting your body from stressed to calm and focused.

ACTIVATING REAL-TIME RESILIENCE

Non-resilient thoughts happen when your brain perceives an adversity as a threat. It's that "itty bitty shitty" voice that tells you that you're not good enough or that you should give up and stay within your comfort zone. It's the thoughts that contribute to stress and trigger the flood of emotions.

The ultimate goal of real-time resilience is to help you change those pesky thoughts so they're more accurate and manageable. You'll learn to have an internal dialogue with yourself in the midst of adversity and perform a reality check.

REAL-TIME RESILIENCE

1. What is another way to view this situation? What is really happening?

2. What's the real cause of this adversity? What is the evidence that points to that?

3. What is the most likely outcome? What's the first step you can do to deal with it?

Answer these questions as honestly as you can, even though it may hurt your ego a bit. One of the pitfalls of using the real-time resilience approach is facilitating illusions of blamelessness and denying any cares or concerns. Avoid unrealistically optimistic beliefs and stick to the facts of the situation. Remember that the goal of these questions is accuracy ("What's really happening?") rather than optimism. Acknowledging the truth in your answers will help you discover a strategy to change it for the better.

Be sure to not play the blame game or depersonalize the adverse situation. Redirecting blame won't help you take control of the situation and you won't be doing yourself any favors in the long run. Don't dismiss the reality of the situation. Being resilient isn't going to make all your problems go away, but it will help you figure out what is the most likely outcome and what steps to take to get there.

The more you practice increasing your resiliency, the better you'll be at it. Understanding when you have underlying beliefs that may be counterproductive or preventing you from focusing on your goals will help you realize when negative emotions are triggered, and the stress is overwhelming. You don't need to give up your quest! Situations that once left you off balance and confused will slowly become history. You'll become more confident and have the inner strength to create the life you want for yourself.

Life can be tricky and unpredictable—there are no guarantees (except death and taxes!). Sometimes, no matter how much you work toward something, you can't figure out why you can't ever reach it. Gaining understanding can be quite a process, and it can make you feel vulnerable and sensitive to every decision you make. Unfortunately, this often leads you to be cautious and defensive instead of willing to try new things.

Your wellness goal must be meaningful enough to challenge old stories and beliefs that hold you captive. When you understand why you want to make changes for the better, it becomes meaningful to you, and you can endure the challenges and become resilient. Bounce back from adversity and obtain better focus by connecting and understanding the meaning in your life! By changing the way you think, you can live a more resilient life and thrive no matter what obstacles you face.

SELF-EFFICACY

Once you build up your resiliency muscle, the next thing to work on is increasing your self-efficacy—the confidence that you can succeed or produce the desired result. Self-efficacy is the belief that you can master your own destiny and effectively problem-solve as issues arise. Having high self-efficacy means that you don't give up when the original solution doesn't work. Instead, you persist until you find a workable answer. In turn, your confidence will increase, and you will persevere through hardships.

People, with low self-efficacy shy away from new experiences because they assume that they're unequipped to meet the challenges. They struggle as they step back and rely on others to search for a solution. Their lack of confidence causes them to give up at the first sign of difficulty, and unfortunately, this becomes a self-fulfilling prophecy. These people will either give up or fail amid adversity, and each negative experience fosters their beliefs that they can't handle any pressure. Not surprisingly, their self-doubt grows, and their worst fears become real.

So, how can we build our self-efficacy? I can tell you what not to do. Pumping yourself with the you-can-do-it platitude, using optimistically enhancing slogans, and having motivational talks really don't do anything. In fact, these things can make it worse. Why? Self-esteem is usually a by-product of doing well in life—meeting challenges, solving problems, and not giving up amidst struggles. When you're struggling, all that positivity is inauthentic. It's not going to make you feel better about yourself, especially when you know the words are empty and untrue.

But how *can* you overcome the doubt of our own abilities to meet the challenges life throws your way? How can you increase your belief in yourself to succeed in a particular situation? How can you develop a stronger commitment and interest in what you're doing and recover quickly from obstacles and disappointments? You need to refer to the four sources of self-efficacy.

SOURCES OF SELF-EFFICACY

Mastery – Performing a task successfully strengthens your confidence. Find a task that you know will be a minor challenge, but that you have a high likelihood of succeeding at.

Social Modeling – Witnessing other people successfully completing a task can help motivate you. If they can do it, so can you! Celebrate the successes of others.

Social Persuasion – Encouragement and positivity from your supporters help you overcome self-doubt and focus on giving your best effort. Surround yourself with positive people who care about you.

Psychological Responses – Moods, emotional states, and stress levels can impact how you feel about your personal abilities in a particular situation. Work on your hobbies, meditate, or find something else that brings you joy and peace.

INCREASE YOUR SELF-EFFICACY

Keep Stretching – We have three personal achievement zones. The "comfort zone," the "stretch zone," and the "panic zone." The trick is to keep yourself in balance in the "stretch zone." Be willing to take reasonable chances and show resilience in the face of failure and setbacks. Setting mini goals for yourself in activities that you enjoy, being open to trying new things, and continually challenging yourself will support your goal to accept your failures as lessons. This will instill your drive to improve constantly. Most importantly, it is wise to approach your goals slowly and not overstress about the results.

Keep Reaching for Small Wins – Build trust in yourself by setting reasonable goals and approaching them one by one, breaking them down into smaller subgoals. Let's say you want to run in a 5K. Your first goal can simply be putting on your running shoes and going on a walk. Next, try to run a couple times a week for ten minutes. Slowly graduate the length and frequency of your runs. Before you know it, you'll be ready for that 5K! By breaking down your goals and feeling success, you'll have the forward movement to encourage yourself to keep at it.

Look at the Big Picture – Let's say you skipped a day and didn't run. That day turns into a couple of days, and then, a full week. Rather than give up on your goal, look beyond the short-term errors and learn from that experience. Did you skip because your body was tired? Did you have a hectic day? Widen your perspective and honor your body by realizing what it can do. When you feel better, get back to it. Self-efficacy allows you to sort out your priorities and create better plan Bs so you can focus on being more effective and efficient with your effort and time.

Reframe Obstacles – Reframing obstacles and adversity can help you reconstruct the way you look at your failures by changing the way you think of yourself. We worked on this a little bit when we discussed the big picture, but let's dig deeper and find ways to positively intervene when you hit an obstacle. Understand and accept that challenges and shortcomings are inevitable—everyone has these. But when you make a conscious choice to continue believing in your strengths and abilities, you will eventually be able to overcome the self-doubt. You will successfully achieve your goal!

One of the techniques I like to use with my clients is the "confidence ruler." When we're designing our strategy plan, I ask them how confident they feel about being able to make this change and meet their goal. When they give me a number, I'll ask why it wasn't lower. They'll proceed to tell me what skills, tools, and abilities they have that increases their confidence level. When I ask them why it wasn't a higher number, we then uncover what they feel that they might be missing. This forces them to see both their strengths and the aspects that could use some work. Often, we'll return to our strategy and incorporate building up those missing pieces so they can find success.

By analyzing at your strengths and weaknesses with an honest eye, you'll be able to incorporate what you're missing as part of your strategy plan. The more you succeed, the more your self-efficacy and resilience will increase. You'll be able to face and even enjoy the challenges that come your way. You may even find yourself looking forward to tackling the difficult tasks because you know that you can overcome them. Self-efficacy will allow you to progress every day, and your increasing belief in your capabilities will help you in all walks of life. You'll be able to sustain your motivation and be more resilient. You'll be able to accept and honor yourself just as you are, gaining strength to follow your goals.

COMMUNITY

Every human is connected to each other, and that connection is important for the well-being and survival of any individual. I recently watched an awards show where the recipient thanked his many supporters who kept motivating him and keeping him on track. It's no surprise this also applies when you are trying to stretch out of your comfort zone and make lifestyle changes. Without a community to encourage, offer advice, and share their own experiences, you will struggle and possibly give up on what you were trying to accomplish. This also connects with the meaning and purpose of your goal. Being part of something bigger than just your own life is a basic human desire. When you're a member of a community, you get to share accountability. It's hard to admit something didn't get done when everyone else has been able to do it.

ADVANTAGES OF A COMMUNITY

Collective Wisdom – Everyone has different experiences, and others' experiences will help you avoid needlessly reinventing the wheel.

That Gentle PUSH – When you're working on a goal on your own, it's easy to give up or sweep it under the rug and forget about it. But when you surround yourself with others working toward a similar goal or objective, you'll get that "kick in the pants" to push yourself just a bit further.

Support and Belief – When things feel impossible, finding someone who believes in you and what you can accomplish can change your story.

Thinking Outside of the Box – Different perspectives and divergent world views mean that we all approach the same problem differently. Melding information from several sources can help find the perfect solution for you.

Inspiration – When you see someone meeting a challenge, most likely you'll be inspired to do the same.

You need to find your community or tribe to help you meet your goals, but how? With technology at our fingertips, it's gotten much easier to find people who align with your own goals and interests. You can download an accountability app, join a group on Facebook or other social medias, or—if you prefer to meet people the old-fashioned way—go to your local gym and make friendly conversation while there to build connections.

It's important to find people who have similar goals and share in your values. For instance, if you're trying to reduce your stress, you wouldn't want someone who has a type-A personality and doesn't understand why everyone else doesn't work as hard as they do. Define your goals—they don't have to be the exact same thing as your tribe but having them be relatively relatable is helpful. Commit to actively participate and make the effort to become connected. Clearly understanding your community's purpose will also help seal the psychological contract with your group.

Make sure you ask each other for updates and don't be afraid to reach out if a member hasn't checked in—this is the purpose of the tribe! Keep the communication simple and easy to follow. Don't ask for a lot of detail, but instead keep the conversation on point. I'm part of a movement accountability group that I found by gathering five girlfriends that wanted to start exercising every day and it has been a game changer for me. I've had chaotic and busy days where I feel too exhausted to do anything, but since I'm obligated to check in, I'll make sure to carve out the time and get on the mat for my yoga session. If I didn't have this group, I would be left to my own devices, and you would likely find me on the couch eating a huge bowl of popcorn instead.

It's also important to be accepting of the fact that you may sometimes come up short of your goals. Life happens, and it's important to keep going despite the setback. There were times that people in my group were dealing with injuries and busy work projects. When they checked in, they received nothing but support and encouragement, which encouraged them even more to make an extra special effort to get back on track. They were able to wipe the slate clean and start fresh, building resilience to reach their goals even when obstacles arose. When you do meet your goal, your community will be your loudest and biggest cheering section, which of course will encourage you to keep stretching yourself and make healthy lifestyle changes!

PACKING CHECKLIST

Whew. . . That was a lot of information!

Now is a good time to see how all of this can apply to you. The following summary and questions should help you put all the puzzle pieces together for your own road trip. I strongly urge you to go through these questions to really understand where you are before you even begin your journey and who you want to be at the destination. These questions will help you understand your why, who, what, and when—notice, I didn't say how just yet. This valuable information will help guide you through your road trip to wellness by showing you what you already have and what you may need to make your trip easier.

I know it may be tempting to skip over this part, but that would be like sitting down to dinner without having cooked it first. When you travel, it's best to sketch out a flexible itinerary. Otherwise, you'd be going in circles with no goals, and this can get frustrating fast. The last thing I want is for you to pack up and call it quits because you don't feel like you're getting anywhere.

Once you get through these questions, your path should become clear. Have fun with the questions, and I'll see you on the other side where we'll focus on the how part of your journey.

REVIEW

DEFINING YOUR WELLNESS

1. What does wellness mean to you? Are your body, mind, and spirit in balance? Does your lifestyle support this?

2. Are you using your full potential? What could you be doing more of? What could you be doing less of?

3. Are you making a deliberate effort to fully realize your wellness?

POSITIVE MINDSET

1. Do you have an open mindset or a fixed mindset?

2. How confident are you that you can change your behavior?

POSITIVE PSYCHOLOGY – PERMA

1. How positive are your emotions? Do you approach things from a positive or negative mindset?

2. Are you engaged in what you're doing? Do you find joy and flow in your daily routine on your way to your destination?

3. How is the quality of your relationships? Do you have people in your life who make you feel like you belong and are valued? Do you feel safe being your authentic self?

4. Can you connect your activities and hard work to a greater purpose or meaning? Do you understand the impact of what you're doing?

5. Do you feel a sense of accomplishment? Have you worked for and achieved a mastery over things that you haven't done before?

YOU ARE HERE

1. Do you really know yourself? Are you accepting of the unique you? Do you appreciate your flaws as helping you achieve your full potential?

2. What are your signature strengths? (Hint – Take the VIA Character Strengths Survey!) How can you use these strengths in your everyday life?

3. Do you know how you work? What did you learn about yourself from the Getting to Know Yourself questionnaire?

4. What did you learn from your Wellness Wheel exercise? What part of your life do you want to work on first?

5. What did you learn from the Vision Board exercise? Who is your future-self?

POSSIBLE DESTINATIONS

What areas do you want to visit first? Why? Don't forget to break these into day trips!

1. Nutrition and Hydration

2. Mobility, Movement, and Exercise

3. Sleep and Relaxation

4. Stress Management

5. Connection

STAGES OF BEHAVIORAL CHANGE

What stage of change are you in? What do you need in order to reach a higher stage? What day trips can you take to support your destination?

1. Pre-Contemplation
   - I won't
   - I can't
2. Contemplation
   - I may
   - I will (preparation)
3. Take Action
   - I am
   - I still am (maintenance)

PACKING CUBES

One of the greatest things invented for travelers are packing cubes. They separate each category of items within your luggage, which is a great concept to carry over to your road trip to wellness.

MEDITATION CUBE

- Is your intention clear? Why or why not?
- How mindful are you?
  - Are you focusing on the past?
  - Are you worried about the future?
  - Are you focusing on the present?
- Do you appreciate the value of the process?
- Can you be less judgmental during this process?

YOGA CUBE

- Avidya
  - Are you recognizing things as they truly are?
- Parinamavada

    - Do you accept the idea of constant change, realize that you're not the same person you were in the past, and that you're constantly learning and becoming someone new?

- Ahimsa

    - Are you practicing love, genuine care, and compassion toward all living beings, and especially to yourself?

RESILIENCY CUBE

- What is your response to adverse situations? Can you change anything to make things smoother?

- What thinking traps can you avoid?

- What are your underlying beliefs? Are your motivations and values getting in the way of responding successfully to adversity? Can you regulate your emotions better and improve your empathy?

- Are you open to viewing the world from a different perspective and not reacting to your emotions? Can you positively change your behaviors when you come upon a roadblock?

- Can you identify genuine threats and see the big picture?

- How do you calm yourself when there are stressful situations? Are your tactics positive? Effective?

- How do you manage that "itty bitty shitty" voice that tells you to give up?

SELF-EFFICACY CUBE

- How confident are you that you can make healthy changes in your life?

- What source of self-efficacy works best for you?

    - Mastery – Practice, practice, PRACTICE!

    - Social Modeling – Where can you watch other people successfully do what you want to do?

    - Social Persuasion – Encouragement and positivity from a support group.

    - Psychological Response – Getting yourself in a positive and relaxed mood.

- How often do you stretch your skills?

- What was the last accomplishment you achieved? Did you break it down to reach that achievement, or did you do it all at one time?

- Did you ever just give up because you didn't think you'd have a perfect record?
- What did you do when you hit obstacles in the past? Did you figure out an alternate path?
- How did you maintain motivation and momentum during this process?

COMMUNITY CUBE

- Who is your support group, your tribe, your community?
- What motivates you the most from a support group?
    - Hearing about their experiences.
    - That gentle PUSH to not give up!
    - Finding people who believe in me.
    - Learning different ideas and perspectives.
    - Watching someone meet the same challenge is inspiring!

SUMMARY

By answering the questions above, hopefully you now understand what you already have and what you need to cultivate. If you felt stuck on some of these questions, you might take a quiet moment to examine your beliefs and feelings and decide to either take it or leave it. We all have different strengths and motivations.

Some people will resonate with this packing list and others will want to bypass the things that make them uncomfortable. It's certainly okay to do the latter, however if you find yourself lost or not heading in the preferred direction, you might want to return to this section and try approaching with a different perspective. If you find that there are many things missing in your packing list, you may want to travel with what you already have and make it a point to visit the destinations that will help you cultivate those missing aspects.

When I was a single mom, I was constantly traveling. I would spend a week at a time with my daughter and then hop on a plane to visit my clients. Clearly, this did nothing to encourage a community for myself and I often felt lonely. I took a road trip to build my community and took specific actions to find and develop my tribe. My life has changed considerably since then, and my tribe has been with me through thick and thin.

By now, you should have a good idea what skills and behaviors you'd like to cultivate. Like a typical adventure, there are no guarantees or hard and fast rules, except to focus on what works for you at the present moment. There's not a single correct answer, as long as you follow your vision.

My intention for this book was to prepare you to be confident in making the lifestyle changes that will improve your wellness. I could have easily made this book three times the length, but I tried to keep it brief. I was attempting to find the balance between being helpful and overwhelming. Hopefully, what you've read so far inspires and motivates you to make the changes to live your life to its full potential, but if you need a little extra help, please look me up in the Resources for Readers section at the end of this book. I'd love to add you to my community and help you grow!

Okay, your suitcase is packed! Now we'll talk about what you should leave behind.

WHAT TO LEAVE BEHIND

"Man cannot discover new oceans unless he has the courage
to lose sight of the shore."
— Andre Gide

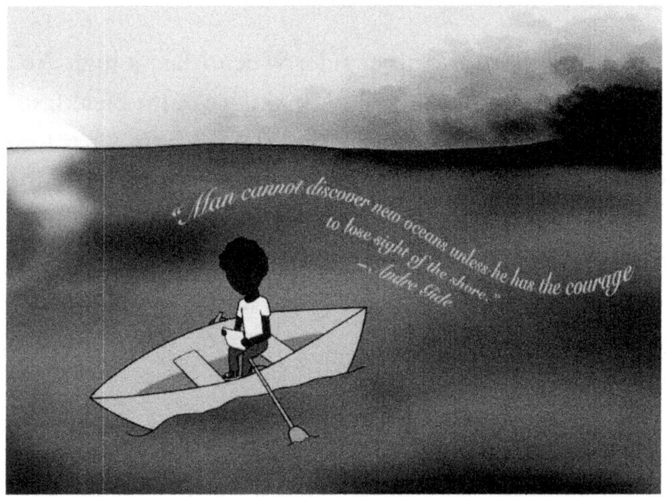

This will probably be the most confusing section. It may seem like I contradict myself often. The truth is, I am. There is no one-size-fits-all path to wellness. You'll have to find a good balance between structure and flexibility. Only you can determine what the right balance is for you, and no matter what your goals are, I'm going to guess that this will be one of your hardest challenges.

Balance has always been a tricky thing for me. All through my life, I've worked hard to get my credentials and have the life I thought I wanted. When I was in the corporate world, I would often work seventy-five hours a week and judge others who didn't put in as much effort as I did. I would eat, drink, and sleep my goals and have complete focus. Unfortunately, when I reached my goal, I looked around to get a high five, but there was no one there. I don't blame anyone. In all honesty, I was not the nicest person when I burrowed in and focused too singularly on the prize.

I've also been on the other side. When I had a high A1C, I really thought that I could just skip cake for breakfast. I certainly didn't plan to make the effort to track what I ate, and because of this, I completely missed the connection of how the few sugary bites I took here and there were affecting me more than I cared to admit. Because I didn't make myself aware of what was going into my body, I didn't make any progress.

As you can see, balance is an important thing. You have to have enough structure in order to truly see how your daily actions and behaviors affect your wellness, but not get so singularly focused that you stress when things don't go according to plan, or you block out any other positive aspects from your life (like connections). It's a tricky dance that you *can* master if you practice enough. Don't let yourself get discouraged when you find your scales out of balance. Simply take a step back to view it with honesty, and then readjust.

RIGIDITY – STRATEGY VS. PLANNING

You've finally made the decision to take action and decrease your stress. You've downloaded the meditation app and signed up for a yoga flow class at your local studio. You're excited and looking forward to exploring this new area in your life—you can already feel the om mantra resonating within your soul. Take that, stress!

Then, you get an important project, which means extra hours. To top it off, you tripped over the dog and fell on your knee, making yoga the last thing you feel like doing. What do you do now? If you're like me, additional stress is already setting in as you try and figure out how you're going to make the project work while hobbling around trying to get your usual tasks done, let alone continue with yoga. Does this sound familiar?

Many times, when we make a goal or try to change our behavior, we experience Murphy's Law—anything that can go wrong, will. Does this mean you have to give up your wellness journey? No! You just need to approach this journey with a flexible strategy rather than a rigid plan.

I used to be very focused, and often had trouble adjusting or modifying my goals when an obstacle arose. This character flaw was not helpful when traveling. In fact, it often took me on a tailspin of constant thinking and obsessing over how my plans were ruined because of life's hiccups. But it doesn't have to be this way!

Being super rigid and strict while trying to change your behavior and adopt healthy alternatives will only lead you to failure. You're learning and adapting to something new. If you let all the obstacles get in your way, you will end up frustrated and even more stressed than ever. You may be completing everything in your plan, but still not seeing the results you wanted. The honest truth is sometimes you can put in 150% and *still* not be where you want to be. No matter how good your performance is, you have to realize that plans have flaws and need to be flexible. Confirmation bias and insanity are both described as doing something over and over and expecting a different result.

It's time to switch your plan into a strategy. A strategy looks outward and focuses on factors that you *can* control. It diagnoses the current situation and your position within it, focusing on the present. Strategy understands that everything is in a constant state of flux, influenced by things you can't control. How you believe that these factors will unfold and shape your success are merely assumptions—you'll need different strategies ready so you can choose which one fits best within what's happening in each moment.

By developing a strategy instead of a plan, you will be more prepared to face the bumps in the road. Because a strategy is flexible, you will develop several plan Bs and have more tools handy to overcome an obstacle. Letting go of what you thought you should do is so much easier when you already have another tactic to replace it. Revising a strategy doesn't mean you were wrong. It just shows that you were aware of unexpected life changes and ready to take them on.

By the way, that example about the big project and wrenched knee. . . Yeah, that was me. I landed a great project right when I had committed to incorporate meditation and yoga into my daily life. Fortunately, by using my strategy and ditching the rigid plan, I was able to integrate both meditation and yoga, albeit in a much different way than my original plan.

I shortened my meditation lessons to very achievable five-minute sessions around mealtimes. I downloaded an online yoga app and started doing ten-minute yoga classes first thing in the morning (to set my morning up) and last thing before bedtime (to decompress and relax). And while I fussed a little as I adapted, I was able to achieve my original goal to reduce my stress level.

It wasn't exactly how I had originally planned it, but the alternatives were pretty darn effective. Side note, I've been doing this plan for the last two years and feeling the results tenfold! Although I had to perform shorter sessions than planned, I was able to get a taste of meditation and yoga, which encouraged me to dive in further when I have more time to spare. My strategy worked when my plan had failed.

TIME MANAGEMENT – FINDING TIME VS. MAKING TIME

Want to know how to get something done? Give it to a busy person.

That sounds crazy, doesn't it? We are so busy in our lives that thinking about changing our lifestyle seems impossible. We're already running around trying to keep our heads above water. Where are we going to find the time to add this extra thing?

The problem is that you will never *find* the time—you have to *make* it. I'm sure your eyes are rolling at this very minute but hear me out. If I were to look for extra time, I would come up empty. Finding time implies that extra time actually exists (if you know the secret behind this, you could probably make a lot of money!). Finding time is like taking advantage of those elusive moments of in-between life. What do you think the odds are of that happening often enough for you to make those changes?

On the other hand, making time is far more deliberate. You have to say yes to something and no to something else. The demand for this time is making you rethink how you spend time in your life. It's choosing what takes priority over other things. When I got overwhelmed with busyness, I stopped myself and made a timecard of my typical day. During stressful days, I realized that I was spending more time stressing about my stressful life—sounds counterproductive, right? To unwind, I spent a lot of time playing games on my phone, scrolling through social media, and reading online news articles. To no one's surprise, this added stress to my day rather than relieving me.

The bottom line is you must prioritize what you want most. I get it—most of the time, we love our lives, and sometimes what we love most is the very thing we probably need to change or modify. For me, I already felt stretched thin, and thinking about adding another thing to my schedule made me very reluctant to change anything. Fortunately, I realized that I was on a treadmill that wasn't going to slow down unless I stopped running. I had to intentionally choose to slow my pace.

My timecard allowed me to see a lot of potential time that could have been put to much better use unwinding in healthy ways. Oh sure, my old habits relieved some stress at the time, but they also created more stress in the long run by putting off the tasks I was stressing about and making me feel guilty for not being productive. By opening my eyes to this catch-22, I was able to make time for activities that were more beneficial and helped decrease my overall stress. I still play games on my phone and look at social media, but it's happily replaced if I have an opportunity to do yoga or meditate instead.

I highly recommend taking the time to jot down what happens during your typical twenty-four-hour day. Include your sleep, meals/snacks, work, and everything in between. Remember, there's no judgment here. You're just gathering information so you can figure out what changes could benefit you. Analyze your card and see if there are activities or behaviors that could be more meaningful and productive. I'm going to repeat: don't judge yourself. Rather, look at your card as an observer. Your soul will tell you what you need the most.

OUTCOME ATTACHMENT – IT'S NOT THE DESTINATION, IT'S THE JOURNEY

The value is in the process. Man, if I could get a dollar every time someone reminded me of this, I would be a billionaire. Despite how annoying this saying is, it's holds so much truth.

One of my clients wanted to fit into her original wedding dress for her tenth anniversary party. We went through the full coaching process from the vision to the reason behind it. We set up destinations and day tours for her to explore, and she was able to create and try different strategies that included eating differently, moving more throughout her day, and managing her stress (she was a self-confessed emotional eater).

Six months later, the day of her anniversary party arrived and she did not fit into her dress. You might be thinking, "Wow, Allie, you must be a TERRIBLE coach!" But. . . wait for it. . ., she didn't fit into her dress because when she got married, she had no muscle tone. At the time of her wedding, she was also stressed out and sick all the time, causing her weight to remain low (and unhealthy!).

Although fitting into her size-four dress was her original goal, she happily told me how great she felt and how everyone complimented her glow. Her newly bought dress showed off her arm muscles, and she felt sexier because she finally had some curves. During the process of trying to fit into her wedding dress, she discovered that she loved ballet. Her love for ballet encouraged her to stick to her eating plan for the energy and strength her new hobby required and gave her an outlet from her stressful job.

You may think you want a certain outcome in the beginning, and this is a good starting point to motivate you to move forward. However, when you get attached to a specific outcome, you can do yourself a major disservice. By only focusing on the outcome, you rob yourself of the joy of the journey. You discount the hard work and effort you expended and fail to appreciate your growth.

In this client's case, she was able to benefit in many other areas besides just wanting to fit into the dress. She felt stronger, healthier, and able to manage her stress. She taught herself how to process her emotions and take time out for herself. She even forgot about her original goal of fitting into her dress! Her sense of worth wasn't attached to the outcome, and the journey itself became exciting and rewarding.

If you find yourself stuck or blocked, check to see if your focus is on the outcome or the journey. Are you fully engaged in the process? Is there a fear of failure in the back of your mind? Are you afraid of what people would think if they knew you failed? Are you so attached to the outcome that you missed out on the journey?

Even in failure, the lessons learned are valuable and will always serve you well. Engaging in the process and putting in your full effort without fear of failure brings excitement, joy, and even success—although, perhaps different from what you originally thought of as success. Awareness of your thoughts and feelings while you're reaching for your goal will give you meaning and intentionality through every step. Ultimately in the big picture, this is the growth and effort worth celebrating—not just fitting into the dress!

ROAD MAPS

"I can't control the wind but I can
adjust the sail."
-Ricky Skaggs

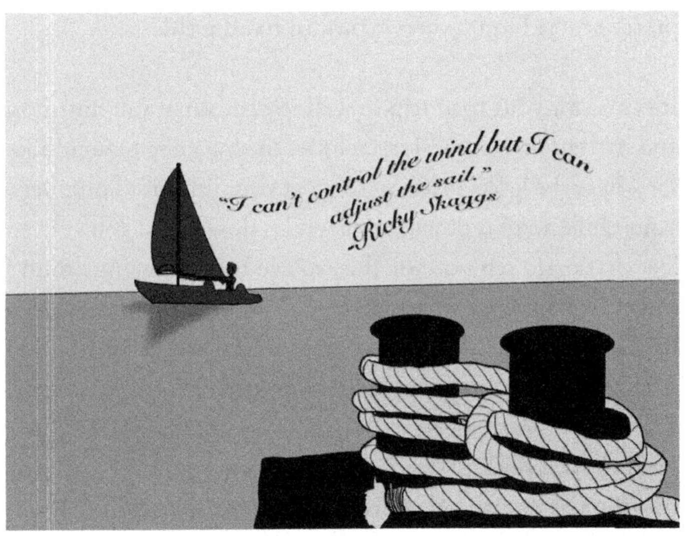

Maps are a very valuable tool when traveling. Sure, it's great to just explore sometimes, but you will need a map to help you pinpoint where you want to go and remind you when you're off target. Likewise, you'll need a map when exploring on your wellness journey, and I hope you'll find these useful!

The common theme here is to break everything down. Smaller goals are less overwhelming and have a higher success rate. Allow yourself to take the journey as slowly as you need to. You aren't doing yourself any favors by rushing it. Rather, this may cause you to feel like your goal is unachievable and just give up.

Let's consider an example. You just got back from the doctor after getting bloodwork tested. The numbers weren't great, and the doctor has told you that unless you can manage those numbers, you'll be at risk for heart disease and diabetes. That's pretty scary! Don't worry, you can handle this.

It's time for your road trip to wellness, destination: nutrition and hydration. Your vision includes the next trip to your doctor where she looks in amazement at your improved numbers. Your cholesterol is down, your A1C is down, and you've even lost that extra ten pounds that you've been carrying around since last Christmas. Best of all, you are feeling fantastic. You have energy you didn't have before, and while life is stressful sometimes, you have it all under control.

How do you achieve this vision? You gain some new skills by reading this book and chart your map to successfully reach your destination. Are you excited yet? Let's get started!

THE VISION

This will be a refresher on setting your vision for your goals and priorities. I can't stress how important it is to start your journey with a clear picture of WHO you want to be at the end of your journey. If you skip this step, you might be wandering around aimlessly. This will result in you missing out on the best thing about traveling—recognizing how much this journey has helped you change and grow.

It's not enough to say, "I want to feel healthier and happier." Unless you can tap into a specific feeling, it's so easy to give this journey up when things get difficult. Your vision is the mental picture of the future you desire. Having a vision will help you prioritize and clarify how you want your life to be and the sacrifices and effort it will take to achieve it. It's kind of like a reality check to set you up for success. We can't all be Tom Brady or Ruth Bader Ginsberg just by wishing. You have to break your vision down into realistic steps to see the process of your dreams turning into reality.

A clear vision can give you a larger picture of your life and reflect changes in behavior to generate the future that you desire. Your passion and dreams will drive and motivate you, but it will require changing your behavior to be able to see and feel what does not yet exist.

It's also important to make sure that your vision integrates with your values and priorities. If these aspects aren't aligned, you will constantly be in conflict. I've seen this countless times in many of my clients. It's easy to focus so strongly on your career and unknowingly sacrifice some of your values on the way to the top. But once you've made it to the top, you won't feel like yourself anymore. In fact, you'll find that you've become a whole different person, but not in the way you wanted. This conflict leads many of us to find distractions or indulge in unhealthy habits to take away this uncomfortable feeling. Fortunately, who you are at the core remains, and it's never too late to make positive changes.

Take a moment to answer the questions below. Let me clarify that there are no right or wrong answers to these questions. This exercise will help you see if your values and vision align, discover your priorities, and prepare for obstacles.

VALUES AND VISION

YOUR VALUES

1. What are the five things you value the most in life?

2. Take thirty seconds to write about the three most important goals in your life right now.

3. What would you do if you won a million dollars?

4. If you only had six months to live, what would your priorities be?

5. What have you always wanted to do, but been afraid to attempt? Why?

6. If you knew you couldn't fail, what one great thing would you dare to dream?

YOUR VISION

1. **Lifetime** – When you look back from your future deathbed, what made you the happiest in your whole life?

2. **Ten years from now** – Who do you want to be? How will you feel? What will your typical day be like?

3. **One year from now** – Who do you want to be? How will you feel? What will your typical day be like?

Are your answers to both sections aligned and connected with each other? If one of the five things that you value is family and connection, but your one-year goal is to get that promotion no matter what it takes, your values and visions aren't aligned. To get that promotion, you may have to sacrifice some family time and focus your efforts at work. More than likely, either your family time or your promotion efforts will suffer because you will continually be in conflict. This will cause you to feel unmotivated and unhappy.

"But Allie, why can't I have both family *and* a career?" You may want to advance your career as well as keep your family connection strong, and I'm not saying that you can't do both, but you will have to find balance. The beauty of this exercise is that you know ahead of time what challenges you will face. Being prepared for these will allow you to come up with a plan B, C, and D to offset the obstacles.

If you find that you're in conflict, you may need to decide what is most important at the present time, and what can be put off until later. Or you might decide that your ten-year goal is so important that a shift in your beliefs is required. Be open to the fact that if your beliefs change, your values may change along with them.

A client of mine had a strong belief that she had to be in charge of everything within her family, her work, and her social group. She ran the house, managed several concurrent projects at work, and often organized social gatherings at her home. Her husband, co-workers, and friends always offered to help, but she would dismiss them. She felt that only she could do it the right way. Needless to say, her stress level was off the charts.

She came to me to develop better sleeping habits—she was averaging four hours a night. She found that she was also gaining weight and her blood pressure became dangerously high. When I took her through these questions, there were a lot of quiet, thoughtful moments. At the end of our session, I asked her what the biggest takeaway was for her. Without hesitation, she said that while she hated having our conversation, she was relieved that we had it.

During our next sessions, we worked on her belief that she needed to control all situations for them to get completed properly. It turns out that the root of this issue was that her immigrant parents put pressure on her to make sure everything turned out as planned. Their motivation behind it is understandable, but it caused an unnecessary lifetime of stress for her. This "do it yourself" mentality was her parents' approach to life as well. My client recalled how small it made her feel when her mother took over her wedding, and when her father died too early of a heart attack.

She wanted different for herself and her family. It became her priority to decrease her stress level and live a healthier lifestyle. She chose to work on letting go of control over certain activities and events and to start practicing self-care activities such as meditation and yoga. She told me it was such a relief to learn how to let go and just let things happen. Her relationships became stronger, she felt less stressed, and her life came into balance.

Let's move into your priorities now and break your vision into smaller behavioral goals.

YOUR PRIORITIES

1. What is your number one priority between the three goals you chose earlier?

2. What steps will this top priority entail?

3. How will you need to change your behavior to achieve that?

DECISIONAL BALANCE

It's not enough to just have a vision. If you never push past this step, then your vision is really a dream—something you wish for, but do nothing about. To make it a reality, you've got to take the steps to achieve it. Break your vision down into baby steps that you can achieve and be consistent with. The hardest part will be admitting honestly how you'll have to change your behavior. You've already done most of the hard work because, if you've read this far, it's clear that your priorities are to become healthier, and knowing that is half the battle!

If you're struggling with discrepancies between your vision and your current behaviors, no problem. I ask the following questions when I want to support my clients in exploring their own discrepancies. Your answers may make you uncomfortable, so please, leave your judgment at the door and take a really hard, honest look at what you want. Do your behaviors support your vision?

List all the reasons that you can come up with to the following questions.

DECISIONAL BALANCE, PART 2

1. What are the benefits of staying the same as you are right now? What value do you get out of your current behaviors? Is it better to just continue on as you are? Why or why not?

2. What are your concerns about staying the same? What are you giving up? Why are you contemplating changing your behavior?

3. What are your biggest concerns about making a change? What challenges will you face? How uncomfortable will you be during the process?

4. What are the actual benefits of making this change? What will you get in return? How important is the value to you?

5. On a scale of one to ten, how good do you feel about all the reasons you came up with?

Reflect on your reasons and motivations. Throw any judgment out the window. Why might you be resistant to making a change? Answer honestly to uncover the true meaning, value, and purpose that would come from making this change.

Let's use some rulers to measure your readiness and confidence. This will assist you in understanding where your mindset is and what adjustments you might need to make. Answer the first three questions on a scale of one to ten, then answer the last two questions with complete honesty.

RULERS

1. **Willingness** – How willing are you to change your behavior at this time? (scale of one to ten)

2. **Confidence** – How confident are you that you can change this behavior? (scale of one to ten)

3. **Readiness** – How ready are you to change your behavior? (scale of one to ten)

4. Why didn't you to pick a lower number? (uncover what you have going for you)

5. What would help you get to a higher number? (uncover what you need to cultivate)

You see where I'm going with this? It's not enough to say you want to lose ten pounds to fit into the dress. You've got to figure out WHY you want to fit into the dress. Is the dress the key, or is it your overall health? Is this something that you want to do because you're feeling pressure from others? Or is it something that you've always wanted, but were afraid of failing? What's behind your fear of changing your behavior? How can you overcome that? Do you really want to change it?

I know that's a lot of questions, but I truly believe most people fail at getting healthy because they don't really understand WHY they want to. If you aren't cognizant of the sacrifices you'll have to make, and you haven't prioritized what you want more than staying in your comfort zone, you are setting yourself up for short-term success or flat-out failure. And let's face it, when you understand the deeper reasons why you want to make a change, you're more likely to be ready to make the necessary sacrifices.

BEHAVIORAL GOALS

Okay, you've checked off all your boxes. You have your vision in mind. You've completed your decisional balance. You've even explored your willingness, confidence, and readiness as well as your motivations for making the changes. So, what's your next step?

Robin Sharma, a spiritual and self-help author, wrote, "A great life is nothing more than a series of days well lived strung together like a string of pearls." This illustrates how our daily behaviors all add up to the life we're living. If our vision is not what we're living right now, then we'll have to change our behaviors to get there!

I have so many conversations with people who love to tell me their vision. You can hear the wistfulness and disappointment with where they're at currently. If you're good at creating a vision, but not so good at executing it, you're living a fantasy. But if you take the time to break your vision down into smaller, easily attainable steps, then you really will get to live your dream.

Let's say your vision is a more energetic you. Someone who's productive. Someone who's more upbeat. Someone who feels better. But right now, it's lunchtime and people are circling your office waiting to talk to you about their issues. Your stomach is rumbling because you ate a candy bar instead of a balanced lunch. When you get home later, you won't have the energy to deal with your family. There's tension everywhere you go, and all you can think about right now is unwinding with a glass of wine and falling asleep in front of the TV. But tomorrow, you will wake up and have to face another day with the same issues.

Feels overwhelming, right? How are you going to even survive the day, much less live your dream? You need to break that dream down and figure out the behaviors that you can eliminate or adopt that would be more in alignment with your vision. It's at this point that most of my clients start the blame game and berate themselves for their current behaviors. I'm going to ask you to not even start on this path. Don't play this game—it's not productive.

The fact that you are here reading this book shows that you want to start on a brighter and healthier path. Now is the time to put on your problem-solving hat and open your mind to different ways to change your behavior. You know deep inside that we're all very different people and the best expert on you is, well, YOU! Be honest with yourself and focus on finding a solution to why your current behaviors may be sabotaging your dream. Explore different behaviors to better support your dream and break it down into baby steps. I've also found that it's best to work backward. Let's test that out using the lunch example from above.

Your behavioral goal is to have more energy. You know if you eat a candy bar for lunch, you'll have a sugar high for the first five minutes, but then it goes downhill pretty quickly! Your day is packed, and you need to get the proper nutrition to give you energy. If you start bringing food to work with you, you'll have it on hand when you don't have time to go buy lunch.

You can always look on the internet to learn what foods are healthy and portable. You also have a lunch cooler that you can start using. You get bored easily, so you're going to need to change up your snacks often. There are some snacks that you're not familiar with. You should try a new one each week to see what you like.

You will start by researching healthy foods. Then you will buy five of the foods that pique your interest and bring them with you to the office and try one new food per week, so you don't get bored. You will always have healthy foods on hand in case you don't have time to buy lunch.

That wasn't too hard, right? I realize I might be oversimplifying this process, but honestly, once you start breaking things down, it's easier to figure out how to change the behavior and determine the steps. Breaking your vision down into the smaller, more attainable steps will help you realize your ultimate vision. It will also build your confidence, increase your self-efficacy, and confirm that you are in charge of your life, not the other way around. Don't worry if your steps are small or seem insignificant. Remember that anything you try (whether it works or not) will keep you moving forward. Following the guidance from the example above, try your own behavioral goal below.

BEHAVIORAL GOAL WORKSHEET

Behavior Goal

____

____

How will you change your behavior?

____

____

____

____

What strengths do you have and what do you need to cultivate to successfully implement this new behavior?

____

____

____

____

Detail the steps to achieve your new behavior.

1. ______________________________________
2. ______________________________________
3. ______________________________________
4. ______________________________________
5. ______________________________________

Are you with me, so far? Let's summarize. You've learned how to break your vision into smaller behaviors that you would like to change. You now understand why you need to do the decisional balance exercise. You've weighed the pros and cons, and ultimately made the decision to take this journey. And you've measured your willingness, confidence, and readiness. You know what you have going for you and what you need to cultivate. You're ready to make some progress! So, what's next?

SMART GOALS

You may have tried setting goals in the past and had difficulty finding success. Goal setting is a common thing, yet at least 50% will give up or have the same goals year after year (think, New Year's resolutions). In most cases, these goals struggle to come to fruition because they are vague, aggressive, or poorly framed. No wonder we give up on undefined, poorly designed goals—they're overwhelming and unachievable.

The solution? SMART goals! Setting a SMART goal will solve these issues by establishing a strong foundation for achieving success. What makes them so SMART? SMART goals are **s**pecific, **m**easurable, **a**chievable, **r**elevant, and **t**ime-based.

Let's use another example to work through the steps to make your goal SMART. You're beginning to rethink your nightly glass of wine and TV time. Although it takes the edge off, it's sort of like the candy bar at lunch time—enjoyable in the moment, but the aftereffects zap your energy and make you feel less than great. Your behavior goal is to change your post-work wind down routine, and that's wonderful!

SPECIFIC

But you need to get more specific if you want your goal to succeed. If you keep it vague, it will be like herding cats (or four small dogs when the mailman arrives). You need to answer the five Ws: who, what, where, when, why.

THE FIVE Ws

WHO – Who's involved in this goal?

Mainly you, of course. But your family is also involved, and usually they want your attention because they don't see you all day while you're at work.

WHAT – What do you want to accomplish?

You want to find a better way to decompress that keeps you feeling great. Falling asleep to the TV after having a glass of wine interferes with a good night's sleep. And there's still tension with your family because you're not connecting with them while the TV is on. If you find a different way to relieve stress at the end of the day, you might improve your relationships with your family members and have more energy for the next day.

WHERE – Where is this goal to be achieved?

At home after work.

WHEN – When do you want to achieve this goal?

ASAP—you need more energy now!

WHY – Why do you want to achieve this goal?

You don't feel satisfied with your typical day. You wake up, work all day, become really stressed, and start it all over again the next day. There doesn't seem to be an end in sight.

Okay, you've established your five Ws. Now, it's time for some follow-up questions.

What specific steps will it take to achieve this?

You'd love to be able to reset yourself when you get home. Also, it would be great to have a family activity to do together. Your whole family is stressed lately, and it seems like they need to burn their anxiety off too.

So far, you're heading in the right direction! But this is still pretty vague—you can't stop here.

How can you make your goal more specific?

You've heard a lot of good things about meditation and how it can reset your day. Yoga might be nice too, but you sometimes get home a little late and don't want the kids riled up right before bedtime. Although, maybe some easy stretching you can all do together could set a nice, peaceful tone for the end of the day. Plus, you don't want the kids to be just like you, finding unhealthy habits to destress. You can all do yoga together, modifying it to fit each of your abilities and teaching your kids how to use healthy habits to unwind.

Bingo! You just made your goal SPECIFIC. You've set yourself up for success with a clear plan in place. So. . .

What is your specific goal/plan?

Instead of drinking a glass of wine and watching TV when you get home, you want to explore meditation and yoga with your whole family.

MEASURABLE

Our next requirement is to make this goal measurable. How will you know if you're making progress unless you make the results quantifiable? Defining the evidence that proves you're making progress will keep you motivated and also help you reevaluate or tweak it if it's not working.

How can you determine your progress in a quantifiable manner? A simple way is to track how many days you don't drink that glass of wine and instead perform alternate calming activities with your family such as yoga and meditation. You could also start tracking how many nights you get quality sleep. It's not enough to simply say that you'll stop doing an unhealthy behavior, you need to commit to this action for a specific number of times per week.

ACHIEVABLE

Your goal should always be achievable. I often have enthusiastic clients who will tell me, "I will just stop drinking wine altogether, and instead meditate and do yoga every day." For the first couple of days, that totally works. However, an expectation to eliminate or master a behavior perfectly the first time out is setting yourself up for failure. You may be able to do it for a while, but most of us will struggle in the long run and end up reverting to our old behaviors.

To make this goal achievable, you need to start small. Perhaps, you try to substitute your new healthy behaviors just two times a week. As you get better and better at this, you can increase your yoga/meditation nights and make them into bigger goals for the next week. The point is you need to make the goal attainable—something that is manageable and allows you to be human.

Another factor to consider is if you have the resources and capabilities to achieve the goal. If not, what are you missing? Have others been able to successfully do this?

Let's break down the yoga/meditation example. What do you need to start meditating and practicing yoga? The first thing is research. Do you have the resources to take everyone to a yoga studio, where things are provided for you and you will have a teacher to guide you? Are there classes you can stream online? Can you find a meditation podcast? Does everyone in the family have a common time to spare for meditation and yoga (soccer practice, homework, social obligations)? The trick to sticking to this goal is to make it attainable and realistic. Work out the kinks before setting the goal so you know how easily you can accomplish it.

RELEVANT

Are your goals aligning with your values and long-term objectives? What is the real benefit attached to your chosen objective? In this case, your goal to switch your wine/TV habit for a healthier stress reliever such as meditation and yoga does connect with your vision of a more energetic you. By eliminating a habit that may sap your energy, you are already on your way to becoming a more vibrant self by getting enough sleep and managing your stress in a more constructive manner.

TIME-BASED

Lastly, a SMART goal needs to have a start date and a finish date. If it's not time-constrained, there'll be no sense of urgency, and you might not take the goal as seriously as if it has a deadline. You could lose your motivation, and this goal may lose its priority status without a defined time frame. The trick to making this goal work for you is to pick an end date that is challenging, but still attainable. (See how everything circles back?)

To recap, let's check to see if this example goal meets the SMART requirements. Instead of drinking wine and watching TV when you get home, you want to explore meditation and yoga with your family. You will start working on this goal on Sunday. Your first week will be to introduce this idea to your family and share the research with them. The second week, you'll try to do this two times, and hopefully work your way up to four times per week by the end of the first month.

S – Is it specific?

Yep, it's specific. It's clear what you will be doing each week, and how you will be changing your behavior. Check!

M – Is it measurable?

You are accountable for the introduction, the research, and the number of times you're putting this new behavior into action each week. Check!

A – Is it attainable?

If your family is willing to try this with you and you start realistically (no headstands or pretzel bends the first week!), meditating and practicing yoga two times a week is realistic. Also, increasing the number of times each week by one is very doable. Check!

R – Is it relevant to your overall vision?

Absolutely! Meditation and yoga have been proven to increase well-being and energy. There is also the added benefit of quality sleep that will give you more energy. Check!

T – Is it timely?

This goal has a definitive beginning and ending. Check!

Congratulations, you have created a SMART goal!

One thing to keep in mind is that you may be continually tweaking your goal. Let's say you give the introduction to your family about starting this new goal, but no one shows interest in joining you. A couple of modifications could be to do it yourself or find another activity that the family might be more interested in and would still meet your criteria of releasing stress in a restful, healthy way. You may decide that you don't like meditating after all. Maybe listening to calming music instead is something that could help smooth that edge and encourage you to relax. There's nothing wrong with adapting to your situation. Just make sure that it's still aligned with your overall vision.

YOUR DAILIES JOURNAL

One of the things that has been a game changer for me is my dailies journal—habits or tasks that you track on a daily basis.

It's so easy for me to say that I'll meditate, take a shot of apple cider vinegar, and work on this book, but if the day is a blur, I can't be sure if it really happened unless it's in my dailies journal.

Tracking these things will help motivate you and keep you accountable. If you're trying a new behavior or habit, the first day is typically easy because your motivation is fresh. But to sustain a new habit over a longer period can be more of a challenge. Let's face it, often we're resistant to the new habit we're trying to adopt because, well, it's new. It's easy to brush it off with an excuse or even to simply forget it because it's not yet an established habit.

You're trying to adopt new routines because you want to improve the quality of your life, and you think that these new actions will be good. Most of us brush our teeth in the morning without even thinking about it because it's good for our teeth and it's part of our daily routine. Why not set up your life to incorporate other healthy habits? A tracking system can motivate you to keep going until your new tasks become a part of your normal everyday routine, especially when life gets a little chaotic.

I find my dailies journal to be very grounding. No matter what crazy thing happens each day, I know that if I make the effort to do my daily habits, I will feel more centered. Having this accountability will help you remember to perform your new habit daily, as well as give you a sense of accomplishment when you look at your journal and realize that you hit your goal five days in a row. Another thought is to write down a brief statement about how you felt before and after performing your new habit.

One of my clients was very resistant to track her new habits. She didn't want to be obsessive and felt that it would be taking all the joy out of her life if she had to constantly record everything. We talked about what might be really going on, and it turns out she was afraid of committing to this new habit. She felt that it would be a downer every time she looked at her journal and saw how she failed to complete her tasks.

You probably can already tell that this client scored low on her confidence and readiness rulers. Believe it or not though, tracking your days will strengthen your commitment to perform these new behaviors, which will in turn improve your confidence that you can make positive changes in your life.

We agreed that we'd leave all the expectations at the door, and for the first week, she was just going to jot down when she remembered to take her daily walk and meditate, not when she forgot. During our check in, she was surprised to note that she walked and meditated three times during the first week. She told me, "I didn't even think about it. I just walked and meditated when it crossed my mind."

I challenged her the second week to walk and meditate three times again. At our next check in, she proudly told me that she meditated four times during the week and walked five times! By the third week, she was committed to walk and meditate five times per week. After three months, she eliminated meditation and walking from her goals because she found that they had become a daily habit for her, and she no longer needed to track them. She now uses her dailies journal for other new behaviors that she's trying to adapt.

People approach personal development in one of two ways—accidentally or intentionally. Most of our motor and social skills happen gradually and unconsciously when we are kids. However, as adults, we mainly grow when we *choose* to grow. It has to be intentional. You are on this road trip to intentionally create healthy habits and increase your wellness. This can be daunting, and unless you track your actions and behaviors, how will you know if you're progressing? If you feel like giving up, you can look in your journal and see how far you've come. This may be just the encouraging push you need in that moment.

Start off by keeping your dailies journal as simple as possible. I made sure at first to meditate and drink my apple cider vinegar. I gradually increased my goals to include tracking the progress of writing this very book and keeping up with functional medicine research. Now my journal is full-blown. I track my fitness, yoga, meditation, work projects, and learning different languages. Keep in mind, I don't try to check all the boxes every single day—that would be insane! Instead, I try for three to four perfect days, and then let the rest go. I also track where I am in each process or what class I take. Often, if I feel run-down and tired, I'll look at my spreadsheet and realize that I worked out ten days in a row! Sometimes, you need to take a rest day.

Your dailies journal can look however you want. You could simply use a calendar and X out each day you fulfill your commitments (there is nothing more satisfying then seeing all the Xs in a row!). Or you can write it in an old-fashioned composition book with the date and what you accomplished. You could also consider an Excel spreadsheet, or there's likely an app out there for tracking the progress of your goals. Find whatever form of a dailies journal that works for you, but start small. Your only objective at first is to include one or two new habits in your routine. Don't obsess the first week—just record when you did the new habit and when you didn't.

For the second week, analyze what you did well and what fell off the radar. Make any necessary adjustments and adapt your goals for this week. Maybe you don't need to walk thirty minutes. Maybe you can start at ten minutes, so it feels more doable. Modifying and adjusting for your busy life is going to help you develop your mindset and establish a routine.

If it's going well, challenge yourself by adding five minutes or a higher frequency for the next week. By sticking to the dailies journal, you'll start to feel a sense of accomplishment, which will motivate you to keep going. You'll feel more control over your life and the weeks won't seem like a blur—you'll know exactly what you did and didn't do, and will be able to analyze why and what you need to change.

Ultimately, tracking your new daily habits and seeing the progress toward your goals will give you a way to have a realistic review of what you're doing over a set period of time. Seeing yourself progress will be a positive addiction that strengthens your focus and commitment. It will give you the opportunity to tweak and adjust to what is happening in your life in each present moment so you can keep moving forward.

EMBARKING ON YOUR JOURNEY

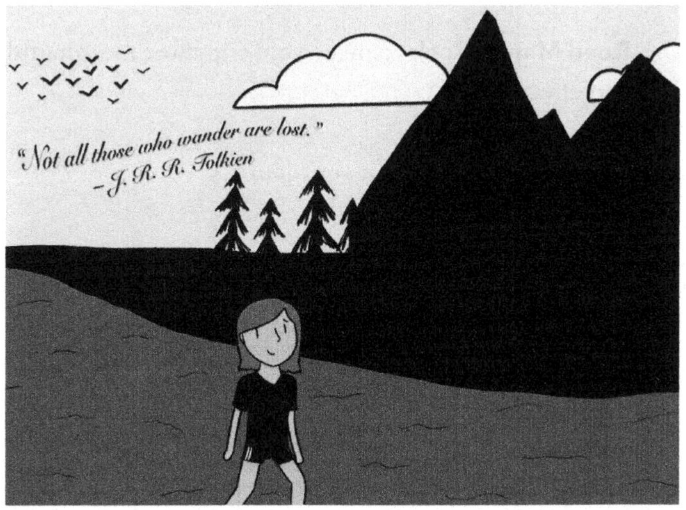

We're in the home stretch! Hopefully by now, you've learned the following things:

Welcome! – Reframing wellness into a road trip

Preparing for the Road Trip – Understanding wellness and cultivating a positive mindset

You Are Here – What you have vs. what you need

Destinations – Choosing your ultimate goals and breaking them down into smaller achievable goals

What to Pack – Essential items for success

What to Leave Behind – They'll only slow you down!

Road Maps – Tools to make your trip more meaningful and effective

Now, it's time to embark on your journey!

DEALING WITH UNCERTAINTY

"I think I forgot something!"

If you're like me, the night before any trip, I lie awake and mentally go over all the details. "Did I pack my toothbrush? Did I pack my bathing suit?" I swear, I forget this last item at least 50% of the time, which is why I have a nice collection of bathing suits! I'm constantly worried that I'm not prepared or don't have everything I will need.

In all reality, you will never be 100% prepared. That's the thrill of traveling or trying something new—you are exploring! The trick is to get comfortable with the unknown, the unexpected, and the mystery of your journey. Reframe your nervous, anxious thoughts into an adventure of new possibilities and experiences. Teach yourself to be open to where your journey may lead.

Many of us are uncomfortable with uncertainty. I certainly am, and that is still on my list as one of my destinations to explore further. Let me share what I have learned so far. The brutal truth is that nothing in your life will ever be a sure thing—life has no guarantees. You can do everything perfectly, and still have the outcomes not be what you expected. You have two choices—you can consistently become frustrated and anxious when things go outside the plan, or you can embrace the mystery and the uncertainty of it all.

There are steps you can take to get better acclimated with uncertainty. The first step is to accept that you don't have ultimate control over your world. Many of us use worrying as a way to predict the future and avoid surprises. You may believe that if you think through every possibility or read everything online, you'll find the perfect solution and be able to control each situation. But as my favorite quote says, "If you want to make the universe laugh, tell it your plans."

Here are four things I learned during my own road trip to wellness.

Refocusing My Mind – What is within your control? You may not be able to control the big things such as the economy or how people act and behave, but you can refocus what is within your control. Mainly, your own actions and responses. By refocusing on the aspects of a situation that you do have control over, you'll bypass endless and ineffective worrying into active problem-solving. No matter what the situation is, you can always decide what attitude and response you will have, regardless of your emotions. It's easy to become overwhelmed by fear and negative emotions, but allow yourself to pause, accept what you're feeling, and find a sense of peace as you deal with the challenges.

Challenge Your Need for Certainty – I got used to being uncomfortable when I realized that I believed if things were not the way I expected them to be, then it was sure to be a disappointment. By believing this, I set myself up to be disappointed a lot! Being stuck on certainty will cause you to miss out on all the good surprises. Many times, being uncomfortable can lead you to unexpected opportunities, new experiences, skills, and exposure to unplanned treasures. One of the things that I've adopted lately is to take up hobbies that I have no natural abilities in. For example, picture the dancing hippopotamus in *Fantasia* when I tell you that I've taken up dancing. I completely suck at it, but I'm having the time of my life and it brings me such joy. Something about the music (and going left when I should be going right) is so liberating. Side bonus—it teaches me to step out of my comfort zone.

Learning to Cultivate Faith – I'm always envious of people who follow religions because I can see their faith as a strength. It gives them something to cling to in times of trial. While I'm not an organized-religion person, there is something to be said about accepting doubt and uncertainty as part of a way of life. We do this in our daily activities—every time we cross a street, get behind the wheel of a car, travel, or meet new people, we're dealing with an uncertain outcome. Our irrational fears and worries tend to be self-generated. There are triggers in our lives that can be prevented by having faith. Focusing on worst-case scenarios or spending time on rumors and half-truths can be avoided if you reduce your exposure to them. You can also recognize when you feel the need for certainty or are craving reassurance and guarantees and look inward to understand what may be happening within your emotions and stories.

Accepting the Present Moment – This was a tough one for me! Often, when I face challenges, I start wishing for the situation to be different. "If only I prepared more. . . If only I didn't hit traffic. . . If only, if only. . ." Focusing on how I wished things were different took much of my energy and made my discomfort even stronger. By accepting the present moment as it is, you will be able to deal with what is right in front of you. It will help you focus on the best thing to do in the exact moment you are in, and in the exact situation you are facing. Why waste all your brain power and emotions on something that isn't real? Strengthening this new mental habit will teach you to deal with uncertainty in a more productive manner.

ENJOYING THE JOURNEY

Comparison is the thief of joy. Become the expert on YOU.

The urge to compare your progress to others will take away much of the pleasure of your own experience. Of course, this is a very easy trap to fall into, and I do this more than I care to admit (even wellness coaches have their off days). However, making comparisons will detract from the value of your journey and often will make you feel like you're failing.

ENJOYING THE JOURNEY CHECK-IN

1. Are you comparing yourself to an unrealistic target? Are you looking at body builders and swimsuit models while trying to lose weight?

2. What are you trying to achieve when comparing yourself to others? Is it to discover tips on how they're succeeding, or does this just ebb away your confidence and self-esteem?

3. What are the positives of your road trip to wellness? Are you improving a skill? Are you learning something? Are you gaining new experiences?

4. Do you feel you aren't enough? Will you really be happier and more content if you gain what others have?

Idealizing somebody else's life because it looks more attractive than yours will grow a spirit of discontentment. Instead, strive to become an expert on yourself. Who are you? Who do you want to be?

BECOMING YOUR OWN ROAD GUIDE

Become the expert on YOU.

DELIBERATE PRACTICE

In her book, *GRIT: The Power of Passion and Perseverance*, psychologist Angela Duckworth explores and examines the approaches of people who strive for continual improvement. Focusing your energy on who you are and what works best for you will help you thoroughly enjoy your life and incorporate positive well-being for the rest of your days. This is the opposite of being complacent with your wellness. Instead, practice like the experts do—this is what we call deliberate practice.

Deliberate practice requires more than just going through the motions, logging hours and hours of work, and never getting the results you want. Instead, it's zeroing in on a narrow aspect of your overall performance. Let's say one of your health goals is to become more fit. You run five days the first week, work too much the second week (you skip all your workouts), and do three workouts the third week. At the end of the fourth week, you feel in worse shape than when you started. No wonder you gave up on this goal!

If you had approached it with deliberate practice instead, you would set your stretch goal. Maybe you want to run a mile in less than fifteen minutes. Rather than just running intermittently and not tracking your pace, distance, or heart rate, you need to focus on your specific weaknesses. Sounds potentially detrimental, I know, but bear with me. Once you understand your weaknesses, you can problem solve and understand how to improve.

FLOWS

There also has to be a balance to deliberate practice. If we live wholly for our road trips and only focus on our deliberate practice, we will forget the joys of everyday living. This is why incorporating flows into your life is incredibly important. Being in the flow means living without constantly thinking about it. It's meeting the present moment exactly where it is and not wanting to change it or let yourself feel bad about it. It's taking each moment as it comes and appreciating all the aspects—the highs and the lows and everything in between. It's being proud of how far you've come and anticipating the excitement of what's on the path ahead.

Flow is being so engaged in your day that you forget you're even doing it, you just do it without dwelling on it. Think about something you're really skilled at and thoroughly enjoy. Maybe it's cooking up a new recipe, solving a math problem, or giving love to a pet. You don't think about it, you just do it. And when you do, your heart and soul sing because you know this is what you were meant to do.

I suggest that you find many flows to keep around you. Sometimes, happiness is elusive, and you will have some sticky interruptions from time to time—that new recipe may turn out horribly, that math problem may stump you, or your beloved pet may pass away. Life is full of many rotating aspects—excitement, frustration, discouragement, persistence, resilience, and challenges. But this is life at its finest. Enjoy every minute by ensuring that you're balancing deliberate practice and flows. Continually stretch for more experiences and lessons that make you feel whole and complete.

RETURNING HOME

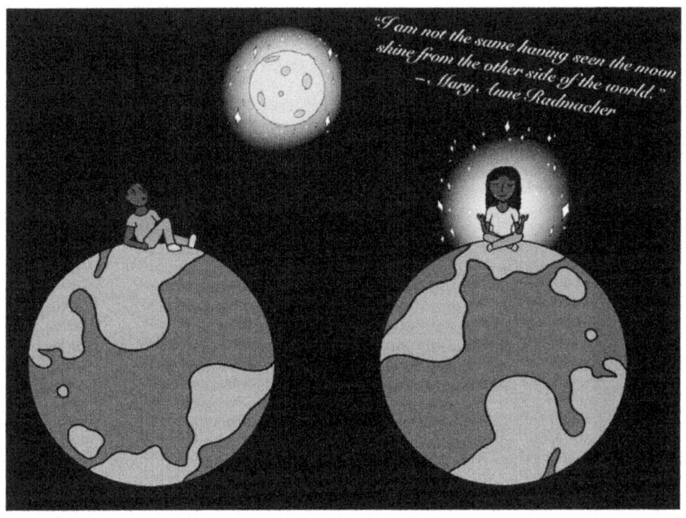

SAVING YOUR SOUVENIRS

I always have mixed feelings when I return home from a trip. I'm so happy to be home and among familiar surroundings, but at the same time, I am wistful for the experiences that I had during the trip. Usually when we travel, we buy souvenirs—trinkets to remind us of our journey and bring those experiences back home with us.

I invite you to think of your new healthy habits as your souvenirs from your road trip to wellness. As you benefit from and continue exploring these new healthy habits, look back and see how far you've traveled to cultivate this healthy new life.

Once in a while, I feel nostalgic and take out my souvenirs to relive the memories. But I've traveled so much that my souvenirs have become disorganized. Some are piled up in the corner of my study collecting dust, and others are tucked away in a closet. This is not ideal for me. I'd prefer to keep my souvenirs front and center to remind myself what I learned and experienced on each journey. I'm going to challenge you to keep your souvenirs front and center after each road trip to wellness.

When you're traveling, it's easy to adopt new habits temporarily because you're in a different environment. Maybe you started walking every morning, or instead of messing on your phone at bedtime, you started reading a new book. You want to be healthy, but you also want to be able to enjoy the pleasures of life. Finding that balance can be difficult, and when you get home, all the same temptations and obstacles that make it difficult to maintain your new healthy habits will be waiting to attack.

Don't worry, I have a solution for you. Remember when we went over the stages of behavioral change? By being aware that you'll have these temptations and temporary relapses, you can prepare and have a plan ready to get you quickly back on track. After your road trip to wellness is over, you will be in a maintenance stage. Hopefully by now, your new behavior has become a habit to the point you perform it almost automatically—at least six months after your initial behavior has changed. Once this transition occurs, you will become highly confident and firmly believe that you've got this handled. And mostly, you do.

However, there's always an Aunt Martha who unintentionally leads you astray. "You must try my fudge brownies! I know you're trying to eat less sugar, but it's just this once" (Aunt Martha doesn't know about the time last week that you gave in "just this once"). Or maybe the day of a big event arrives, and you're busy getting ready, enjoying it, and then recovering. Suddenly a week later, those morning yoga sessions have disappeared, you can already feel stress levels rising and your body responding to the lack of movement.

Does any of this sound familiar? It's okay, you're in good company. It's an unfortunate guarantee that relapses will occur. You will have moments where you temporarily abandon your new behavior that you fought so hard to gain. But the good news is you are a different person now. You can find support to help you regain your focus on the vision you've created. You have the proper tools in your toolbelt to help you take the right steps to return to your healthier lifestyle. You've gained awareness and resiliency. And you've experienced firsthand the benefits and value that these habits can reap. This time around will be a lot easier.

DEALING WITH RELAPSES

The first thing you need to do when a relapse occurs is to reconnect with your strengths, values, resources, visions, goals, and motivations. Remember to remain judgment-free and understand that this is just part of the process. It's life's way of reminding you to listen and reflect, approaching this challenge with curiosity and unraveling it bit by bit.

The next thing to do is enlist support. Find people who are doing the same things that you want to continue doing. Join a studio, find a diet buddy, enlist your family to be your accountability partners, or start a journal. This may also be a good time to hire a coach (Hi!) to help you reconnect with why you wanted to make this change in the first place!

And finally, set up tangible rewards for yourself. Do something small and enjoyable at the end of the day when you've met all your goals. I reward myself with a foreign movie—it makes me feel like I'm traveling in my own home! Maybe for you, the reward could be a visit to the nail salon, a glass of wine, or a long, hot bath. Find something that motivates you and excites you—bonus points if the reward is as healthy as your new goals!

EMBRACING FEAR AND FRUSTRATION

Someone once asked me if I was truly happy. I admit, I had to think about my answer for a bit. And then the meditation lesson of impermanence came to mind. Nothing is ever permanent, which means nothing will ever stay the same. This includes my emotions and moods, the good times and the bad times. That's the beauty of life, and when we accept our present moment as it is, we find inner peace.

My answer was, "Yes, I'm truly content." I know there will be steep mountains to climb and deep valleys that I'll slide down on occasion. I know I may struggle and then triumph or triumph and then struggle. But the one thing that I can count on is who I am on the inside, and that is what traveling has done for me—it's put me in situations that were unfamiliar, thrilling, scary, and dazzling all at the same time. It's taught me that I can overcome my fears, I can build my resilience, and I can achieve my goals.

The traveler's spirit is vital for any road trip, especially your wellness journey. A traveler must learn to eagerly look forward to life's challenges and embrace the fear and frustration of the unknown. In Pema Chodron's book *When Things Fall Apart: Heart Advice for Difficult Times*, she writes, "When you can smile at fear, there's a shift: what you usually try to escape from becomes a vehicle for awakening you to your fundamental, primordial goodness, for awakening you to clear-mindedness, to a caring that holds nothing back." Fear awakens your mind.

Chodron tells a story about a young warrior who had to battle against Fear. She was apprehensive and resisted at first, but her teacher said that she must do it. The day of the battle came. The warrior stood on one side, and Fear on the other.

The warrior asked, "How do I defeat you?"

Fear answered, "My weapons are that I talk fast, and I get very close to your face. Then you get completely unnerved, and you do whatever I say. If you don't do what I tell you, I have no power. You can listen to me, and you can have respect for me. You can even be convinced by me. But if you don't do what I say, I have no power" (Chodron, *Fall Apart*).

In that way, the warrior learned how to defeat Fear. If you avoid what's uncomfortable and let your fears intimidate you, you'll never know your capacity to overcome those fears. Alternatively, if you allow yourself to respect and feel your fears, you can reframe it as a catalyst to work on yourself. By cultivating your strengths to defeat those fears, you will emerge as the victor.

The same thing has been said about frustration and anger. I am prone to irritation and easily annoyed. I find if I don't address it, it becomes full-fledged repressed anger. For me, this is collectively caused by LA traffic, a dog incessantly barking at everything that moves, phone calls or texts coming every five minutes, and loved ones who unknowingly interrupt during a deep state of focus and production. If you can imagine a big, dark red fiery ball stirring inside of me, you know what I can feel during all of that.

I listened to a wonderful meditation on the Insight Meditation app by Alexandra Love where she discussed anger. She talked about how to reframe angry feelings as a warning to ourselves that something needs to change. Instead of trying to repress, ignore, or act out when we have these feelings, learning to embrace them is a much more productive way to manage the little irritations that find their way into our daily lives.

I tried implementing her methods recently and—believe it or not—it works! I use the knowledge of my triggers and adapt my routine to compensate for them. I started using Amazon's Audible to distract me from the stop-and-go of traffic. I close my office door to both the dog and family members when I am working. I silence notifications on my phone when I need quiet thinking time. As a result, I feel less irritated and can better enjoy my time with family after getting in a successful workday in my distraction-free work zone.

If you're bickering with your family, it could be a sign that you need to sit down and set some mutual ground rules. If you're constantly frustrated because you're exhausted and not getting enough sleep, it could be a good idea to aim for an earlier bedtime. If you're grumpy and snap at others after lunch, it could be time to pass on the candy bar and incorporate more nutritious foods into your meals. Listen to yourself. Look at your frustration and impatience as tools to make positive changes in your life by either accepting, modifying, or eliminating those irritations. If you embrace these moments as opportunities to learn and grow, you may be able to change your perspective.

THE ETERNAL TRAVELER

Some people lay awake the night before a trip and anxiously go over everything that can go wrong. Rather than being excited for the adventure, they become resentful of the event that's interfering in their comfortable routine. Boy, do I understand this perspective. When my daughter was young, I traveled every week for work. It was a constant battle to make my flight connections, pack the right shoes (believe it or not, one time I packed a navy blue and a black pump as a pair—I learned never to pack in the early morning!), and have enough energy for my daughter when I came home at the end of the week.

Traveling is tough. It forces you out of your comfort zone. Even when you know where you're going and what you're striving to do once you get there, the anxiety can set in without much effort. You never know if you'll miss your flight, have to scramble because your hotel mixed up your reservation, or if you'll get lost in an unfamiliar area. The energy you expend to deal with all these unexpected occurrences can wipe you out.

Similar to traveling, working toward increasing your wellness can be intense. It forces us out of our comfort zone and adds the stress of the consequences that can happen if we don't reach our goal. The energy we expend to deal with all the unexpected blips can make us feel discouraged, stressed, and lost.

Fortunately, we can change our perspective with a few tweaks. I now find traveling to be intoxicating. Although the trips can still sometimes be rough, if you mention a trip to me, I'll mentally start planning my itinerary and thinking about what I'll need. I love the idea of visiting somewhere new and having different experiences from my normal routine.

So, how can we offset challenges? By making sure we shift from a fixed mindset to a growth mindset. Your mindset can change the way you think about yourself, for better or worse. It affects the way you feel, what you're capable of achieving, how you'll meet challenges, and whether you're open to developing new beliefs, attitudes, and skills. Acknowledge and respect your fears, but don't let them have power over you. Learn to highlight the positive aspects and view the negative ones as opportunities for new experiences and growth.

Dr. Carol Dweck had always been intrigued how some people persevere while others in identical situations give up. She pursued this question throughout her career and published her findings in her book, *Mindset: The New Psychology of Success.* In her book, Dweck discusses how much your mindset, whether fixed- or growth-based, can affect your outlook and have great effects on your entire life.

A fixed mindset believes that talent and intelligence are static and can never change. This leads to hiding flaws and mistakes, feeling ashamed about things that don't work out, giving up easily, and being unmotivated to strive for anything except the status quo. A person with a fixed mindset will avoid challenges to prevent the possibility of failure. They believe that talent is pure luck, therefore effort and practice are unimportant. They view temporary setbacks as permanent failures, which leads to negative feelings such as guilt, inertia, and isolation. A fixed mindset causes people to feel threatened by the success of others. They will ignore constructive criticism because they view it as useless negative feedback. Consequently, they will plateau early and never reach their full potential.

On the other end of the spectrum, someone with a growth mindset embraces challenges and lifelong learning. They recognize that setbacks are a necessary part of the learning curve and see shortcomings as temporary and changeable, maybe even a challenge to try harder. They believe that skills, talents, and knowledge can always be improved, and will therefore put in more effort. They believe that effort leads to mastery, and they will continue to grow throughout their entire lives with open minds. People with a growth mindset welcome feedback and glitches as opportunities to learn and are inspired by others' successes. They understand that not being good at something is a temporary state. Rather than feeling bad or ashamed when things don't happen as planned, they reach further and stretch to their full potential.

Your journey to wellness requires a growth mindset. (Don't worry if you feel you are part of the fixed-mindset camp. You can take control and change this!) Wellness must be developed and demands a strong desire to learn more about yourself and your body. It asks you to persist in the face of setbacks (like when you eat three pieces of pie for dinner) and finds lessons and inspiration from your mistakes (if you have trouble resisting, don't buy the whole pie—buy individual pieces!). And remember, this is a journey, a process.

After you travel, you should have developed a new growth mindset as you broaden your perspective and realize things can be different—life is meant to be fluid, not stagnant. A growth mindset will teach you to enjoy your life as it is, but also be motivated to reach your full potential.

During your wellness journey, you will learn alternate approaches and value the new experiences over your daily routine. You will learn to live in the moment and minimize concern about the past and future. Freeing yourself from your self-made prison, you will become independent and an expert on you. You will gain confidence in your abilities and future potential, purposely leaving your comfort zone and becoming more flexible and adaptable, often even embracing the unexpected. These new opportunities will whet your appetite to explore more ideas and cultures. You'll become a more creative problem solver and see the world as a source of inspiration. With a newfound confidence, you will take the time to build up good habits and work on yourself to become more resilient and open to challenges.

As you put this book down, I hope you have been inspired to take your own road trip to wellness. By now, you should understand what wellness means to you, know where you are in the behavioral change stages, and have opened your mind to make those healthy modifications. Knowing where you're starting from will help you honor yourself by using your strengths and unique process to implement the new behaviors. You've set your vision and have chosen to explore healthy variations that will enrich your life. You've brainstormed projects, experiments, and new habits that will make you feel good, and prioritized which ones you'll check out first.

You're packing your intentions, mindfulness, philosophies, and resiliency to make your journey more meaningful and comfortable. Leaving behind old ideas and bad habits, you're using your new road map to help you set goals and priorities. You've assessed your readiness and figured out what it will take for you to succeed. You've set SMART goals so you can track your progress and figured out exactly how to implement these goals into your daily life. You're ready to take this trip and deal with the uncertainty, striving to become the expert travel guide of your own life and pursue your own unique experience. You're ready!

We're at the end of this journey, my friend. I hope you feel more confident about achieving your vision, and I wish that you will find joy in the journey. Your souvenirs from each trip will allow you to embrace the fear and frustration that comes along with future trips and remind you that you can succeed. Your new growth mindset will inspire you to continue growing and enjoying life to the fullest.

WELCOME TO THE CLUB OF ETERNAL TRAVELERS!

"Twenty years from now you will be more disappointed by the things you
didn't do than by the ones you did do. So throw off the bowlines, sail away
from the safe harbor. Catch the trade winds in your sails. Explore. Dream.
Discover."
–Mark Twain

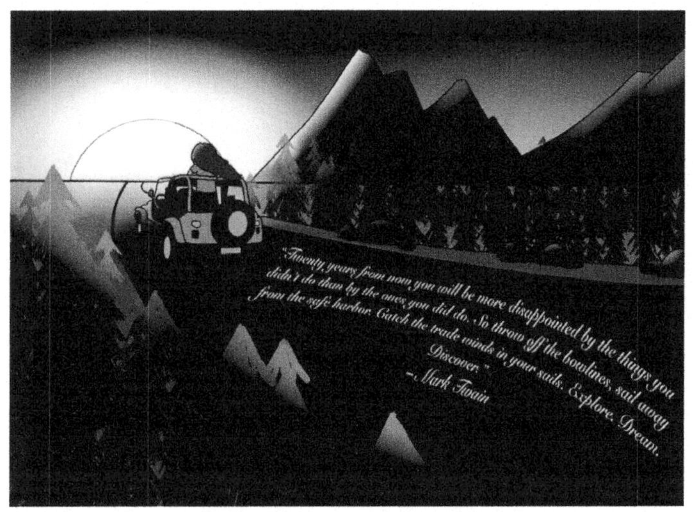

BON VOYAGE!

ABOUT THE AUTHOR

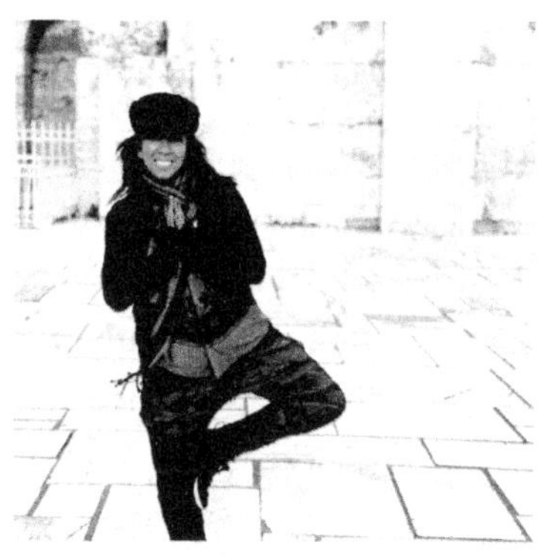

Allison "Allie" Lowe is a National Board-certified health and wellness coach, yoga and meditation teacher, and author of *Your Road Trip to Wellness: A Travel Guide to Making Lifelong Lifestyle Changes for a Happier and Healthier You!* Allie is also the founder of Ready, Set, Go!, a lifestyle management coaching firm, and enjoys helping her clients live their best lives and reach their full potential.

After getting her MBA in organizational learning, Allie spent over twenty years as an executive recruiter and consultant, where she helped people achieve their career dreams. She led and developed change management teams by establishing benchmarks, goal definition, timelines and milestones, and monitoring progress. During this time, Allie honed her strengths with contingency planning.

In 2016, Allie began her own road trip to wellness. She acquired her certification as an integrative nutrition and functional medicine coach, as well as her national certification in yoga and meditation. Allie discovered her sweet spot was helping clients understand, define, and visualize what makes them happy and healthy. She loves the challenge of removing obstacles, energy drains, and clutter. At their own pace, her clients accomplish what they set out to do while overcoming their fears and anxiety to create positive, meaningful experiences for themselves.

Allie is an avid traveler and will mentally plan a trip in her head when someone mentions their desire to travel. Her top character strengths are love of learning, curiosity, and creativity, which means you will always find her learning something new, asking a lot of questions along the way, and finding a workaround for every challenge. Allie hopes to age gracefully and is gleefully delighted when people mistake her for her daughter's sister. Allie is also an animal shelter foster failure and would have over a hundred dogs if her partner, Chris, would allow it.

Allie firmly believes that anyone can accomplish everything they set out to do using the following principles:

- Life is about the journey, not the destination.
- The value is in the process.

- Deliberately practice, and then let it flow.

- You have choices!

Using these principles, Allie has been able to guide her clients to connect the dots between where they're starting from and who they want to be. She loves helping them craft their own personal blueprint and discover their unique needs. All these elements assist her clients to set personal goals, work toward sustainable changes, and live the life they always dreamed of. Allie believes you can succeed also!

ACKNOWLEDGMENTS

Writing a book has been a lifelong dream of mine. Now that I've accomplished my goal, I'd like to recognize the people who have made an impact on my journey and given me the support and encouragement to write this book, as well as the great leaders and teachers who inspired me on my own road trip to wellness.

My Teachers:

Steve Borek, MCC, PMC, BCC, MBA – Steve taught me one of my underlying principles: "the value is in the process." He also inspired me to go after my dreams, and I hope he's enjoying his time in SE Asia, coaching and inspiring people worldwide to find their endgame.

Joshua Rosenthal, founder of the Institute for Integrative Nutrition – Joshua's organization started the engine for my own road trip to wellness and fueled my passion for understanding why we make the food and lifestyle choices that we do.

Dr. Mark Malek – Mark's encouragement and specialty in functional medicine steered me to studying it as well. With an in-depth look at integrative, holistic medicine, I discovered how we can approach our health with positive results.

Dr. Sandra Scheinbaum, founder of the Functional Medicine Coaching Academy, Inc. – Sandra's academy gave me the foundation to help my clients in a positive, effective, and compassionate manner.

Dr. Angela Duckworth, author of *GRIT: The Power of Passion and Perseverance* – Angela's research, books, and concepts have helped me understand the beautiful combination of passion and long-term perseverance.

Tiffany Cruikshank and her wonderful organization, Yoga Medicine – Tiffany taught me so much about myself, my body, and my brain through a yoga lens. Her teaching team, Valerie Knopik, Allie Geer, Diane Malaspina, Megan Kearney, and Brie Galicinao, continually inspire me on and off the mat.

Chandler Bolt and his super-charged, supportive team at the Self-Publishing School, with a special mention to Kerk Murray – The SPS team has made this challenging hill easier to climb, helping me unravel the mystery of writing a book. Their constant support and gentle prodding have made my lifelong dream come true!

My clients – My clients have been the greatest teachers of all. They have been vulnerable, courageous, and inspirational. I'm so grateful to them for agreeing to share their stories so that other people will know that success is around the corner!

My colleagues and tribe have enriched my wellness journey and made it fulfilling. I'm incredibly grateful to have them in my life, constantly learning and laughing alongside me. With them, I'm ready to take on any journey that comes across my path.

My Colleagues and Tribe:

Dr. Lindsay Broderick, DO – Lindsay, you and I have been friends forever and have watched each other grow and blossom. Thank you for your eternal support and the candor and honesty that makes me go to you first when I need to figure things out!

Kate Motz, NBC-HWC – Kate, getting to know you virtually for two years in class is not the usual start to a great collaboration. However, I love that we found a way to connect anyway, and by the time we got to meet in person, I knew right away that you were a forever friend. It was your courage that inspired me to write my own book, and I thoroughly appreciate each of our Zoom catch-ups.

Jess Cherne – Jess, you have such talent with articulating and creating images from my brainstorms. Thank you for your patience and diligence. I still think you should change your major!

Sara "Gracie" Brounstein – Gracie, you've truly been my travel partner during the best years of my life. With you by my side, I've laughed, learned, and loved because of your existence. I can hardly wait to see how our journeys unfold.

Chris Krummell – Chris, my sweetie pie forever, I'm so grateful and honored that we get to travel through life together. Thank you for your support and love. Here's to our next adventures!

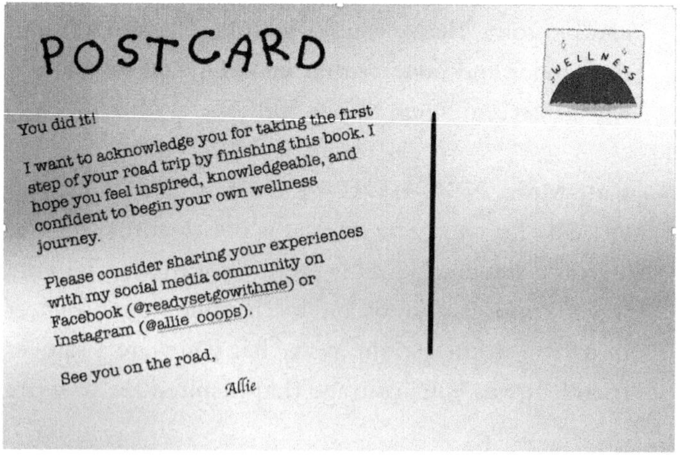

RESOURCES FOR THE READER

WITHIN THIS BOOK

- **YOU ARE HERE**
    - Character Strengths (informational)
    - Getting to Know Yourself (exercise)
    - The Wellness Wheel (exercise)
    - Setting Your Vision (exercise)
    - Vision Board (exercise)
- **DESTINATIONS**
    - Destinations (informational)

  - Decisional Balance (exercise)
- **WHAT TO PACK**
  - Clear Intention (exercise)
  - Thinking Traps (informational)
  - Thinking Traps (exercise)
  - Challenging Your Beliefs (exercise)
  - Problem Solving in Adversity (informational)
  - Calming Techniques (informational)
  - Real-Time Resilience (exercise)
  - Sources of Self-Efficacy (informational)
  - Increase Your Self-Efficacy (informational)
  - Advantages of a Community (informational)
- **ROAD MAPS**
  - Values and Vision (exercise)
  - Decisional Balance, Part 2 (exercise)

- Rulers (exercise)
- Behavioral Goal Worksheet (exercise)
- The Five Ws (exercise)
- Enjoying the Journey Check-In (exercise)

- **RETURNING HOME**
    - Dealing with Relapses (informational)

OUTSIDE THIS BOOK

- VIA Survey of Character Strengths, www.viacharacter.org/survey
- Ready-Set-Go! with Allie Lowe, http://www.ready-set-go.me
- Facebook, @ReadySetGoWithMe
- Instagram, @allie_ooops

RECOMMENDED READING

- *A Seeker's Guide to the Yoga Sutras: Modern Reflections on the Ancient Journey,* Ram Bhakt

- *GRIT: The Power of Passion and Perseverance,* Angela Duckworth
- *Mindset: The New Psychology of Success*, Carol S. Dweck, Ph.D.
- *Positive Identities: Narrative Practices and Positive Psychology,* Margarita Tarragona, Ph.D.
- *Social: Why Our Brains Are Wired to Connect,* Matthew Lieberman
- *The Heart of Yoga*, T.K.V. Desikachar
- *When Things Fall Apart: Heart Advice for Difficult Times,* Pema Chodron

BIBLIOGRAPHY

Chodron, Pema. *When Things Fall Apart: Heart Advice for Difficult Times* (Boulder: Shambhala Publications, Inc., 2016).

Desikachar, T.K.V. *The Heart of Yoga* (Rochester: Inner Traditions International, 1995).

Duckworth, Angela. *GRIT: The Power of Passion and Perseverance* (New York: Scribner, 2016).

Dweck, Carol S., Ph.D. *Mindset: The New Psychology of Success* (New York: Ballantine Books, 2016).

Institute on Character. "The VIA Character Strengths Survey." Accessed April 6, 2019. https://www.viacharacter.org/account/register

Lieberman, Matthew. *Social: Why Our Brains Are Wired to Connect* (New York: Crown Publishers, 2013), 43.

Mead, Elaine, BSc. "The History and Origin of Meditation." Published May 18, 2021. https://positivepsychology.com/history-of-meditation/

Merriam-Webster. "Journey." Accessed April 6, 2019. https://www.merriam-webster.com/dictionary/journey

Merriam-Webster. "Wellness." Accessed April 6, 2019. https://www.merriam-webster.com/dictionary/wellness

Peterson, Christopher, Ph.D. "What Is Positive Psychology, and What Is It Not?" Posted May 16, 2008. https://www.psychologytoday.com/us/blog/the-good-life/200805/what-is-positive-psychology-and-what-is-it-not

Seligman, Martin E.P., Ph.D. "Positive Psychology: Martin E.P. Seligman's Visionary Science." Online course. Accessed June, 2019. https://www.coursera.org/learn/positive-psychology-visionary-science?specialization=positivepsychology

Spector, Nicole. "Smiling can trick your brain into happiness – and boost your health." Updated January 9, 2018. https://www.nbcnews.com/better/health/smiling-can-trick-your-brain-happiness-boost-your-health-ncna822591

Tarragona, Margarita, Ph.D. *Positive Identities: Narrative Practices and Positive Psychology* (San Bernardino: Positive Acorn, 2014), 1.

The Free Dictionary, medical dictionary. "Wellness." Accessed April 6, 2019. https://medical-dictionary.thefreedictionary.com/wellness

The Lancet Global Health. "Global, regional, and national estimates of the population at increased risk of severe COVID-19 due to underlying health conditions in 2020: a modelling study." Published June 15, 2020. https://www.thelancet.com/pdfs/journals/langlo/PIIS2214-109X(20)30264-3.pdf

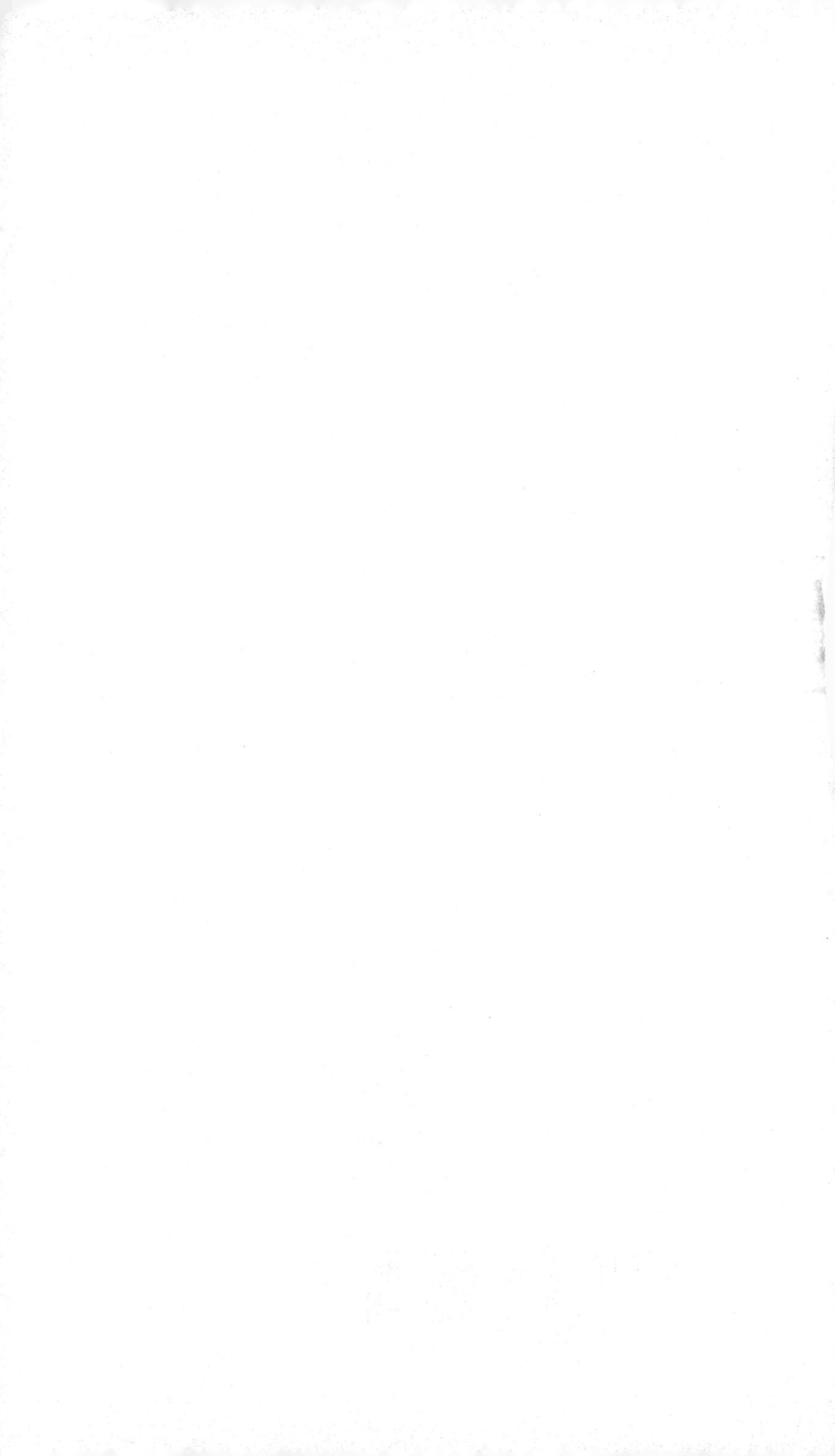

Made in the USA
Middletown, DE
14 May 2022

65638293R00146